ENHANCING FERTILITY NATURALLY

ENHANCING FERTILITY NATURALLY

*Holistic Therapies for
a Successful Pregnancy*

Nicky Wesson

Healing Arts Press
Rochester, Vermont

Healing Arts Press
One Park Street
Rochester, Vermont 05767
www.InnerTraditions.com

Healing Arts Press is a division of Inner Traditions International

*Note to the reader: This book is intended as an informational guide. The remedies,
approaches, and techniques described herein are meant to supplement, and not to be a
substitute for, professional medical care or treatment. They should not be used to treat
a serious ailment without prior consultation with a qualified health care professional.*

Library of Congress Cataloging-in-Publication Data
Wesson, Nicky.
    Enhancing fertility naturally : holistic therapies for a successful
pregnancy / Nicky Wesson.
        p.   cm.
    Originally published : London : Vermillion, 1997.
    ISBN 0-89281-832-8 (alk. paper)
    1. Pregnancy. 2. Childbirth. 3. Infants (Newborn)—Care. 4. Holistic
medicine. 5. Alternative medicine. I. Title.
RG525.W567   1999
616.1'7806—dc21   99-13567
                                            CIP

Printed and bound in Canada.

10 9 8 7 6 5 4 3 2 1

This book was typeset in Helvetica and Century Old Style.

CONTENTS

ACKNOWLEDGMENTS

I am grateful to everyone who helped me to write this book, especially all the people who talked willingly to me about their personal experience of infertility, a private and sensitive subject; their help was invaluable. I would also like to thank Linda Carpenter and David Raitt, without whom my task would have been impossible, and the following: Angela Yates, Heather Guerini, Jill Nickalls, Jill Cook, Adrian Stoddart, Christine Hall, Christine Grabowska, Robert Low, Sue Francia, Jo Kaplan, Ann Kenefeck, Ros d'Albert, Denise Tomlinson, Roy Kelly, Royal Society of Medicine Library, Chris Bell, Caroline Casterton, Anna Knight, Helen Stapleton, Dian Mills, and Lesley Axelrod.

INTRODUCTION

Subfertility is a relatively common problem but, because it is one that strikes deep into the psyche of couples who experience it, it is often concealed, so that it is far more common than is generally realized. It is estimated that as many as one in six couples have difficulty in conceiving the number of children they want when they want them.

In the past and until quite recently, people had little real control over their fertility and couples who did not become pregnant when they wanted a family could do little but accept it. Although it was undeniably hard for them, they had no alternative and they could not reproach themselves for it or for not doing more to overcome it. Nowadays there is more hope for people in this situation, but with hope comes the prospect of treatment stretching out interminably, perhaps involving invasive, embarrassing, costly, damaging, and humiliating procedures which may or may not work. Of course, if the treatment is successful it will all seem worthwhile, but it may be harder to carry on in hope—with tantalizing possibilities always arising however minimal the success rate—than it may have been in the past. The end point can stretch ever further into the distance, with people being unable to accept their situation unless every possibility has been investigated.

One of the aspects that people who have had difficulty in conceiving dislike most is their feeling of lack of control. They also complain of feelings of isolation, depression, and an inability to tell others about their situation or discuss it with them. They find that, when they do, people make comments that seem unhelpful. They are vulnerable and may perceive medical help as being their only way forward. They may feel that there is little that they can do to help themselves, their only chance of parenthood depending on having their condition medically assessed and diagnosed and accepting medical or surgical treatment.

Many people are helped in this way and are grateful to their doctors for assisting them. However, around a quarter of couples who have not become pregnant after twelve months of unprotected intercourse (the definition of subfertility) will find that there is nothing apparently wrong with either of them and, as far as diagnostic tests currently available are concerned, the results of their tests are normal. In such cases of "unexplained," or "idiopathic" or "functional" infertility, couples may be advised that nothing can be done to help them. In fact, both for them and in some cases where there is an apparently over-whelming and insurmountable barrier to fertility, such as blocked tubes, there are effective steps they can take to over-come their problems. These measures, some of which involve simple changes in lifestyle, and others which involve the use of alternative or complementary medicine, can give control back to couples and improve their health and general well-being, and may help them to have a baby. For example, it has been proven that relatively moderate caffeine consumption both delays and reduces a woman's chances of conception. Although women who drink a lot of coffee, tea, and cola do become pregnant, those with borderline fertility may not.

Moreover, alternative therapies have helped many couples to have the children that they so wanted. Because infertility is such a sensitive subject, many couples who have used these methods successfully prefer to keep it to themselves. For this reason, combined with the lack of published research on infertility and complementary medicine, its efficacy may be either unknown or underestimated. However, as the stories in this book show, plenty of couples feel that it has been effective for them. They believe it has worked by restoring them to health generally so that they started to function well and became fit for pregnancy or fatherhood. Specific imbalances or areas of ill health were corrected so that their entire bodies became stronger, rather than particular organs being targeted and forced into action in isolation (as may occur, for example, when drugs to induce ovulation are employed).

Drug prescription, even when effective, removes conception from the intimate relationship between partners and means that it is to some extent beyond their control. Besides this loss of control, there are drawbacks and disadvantages to all forms of medically assisted conception, and some of them have potentially serious long-term effects. Many couples would prefer to avoid these risks—if they realized they had a choice, or knew alternatives were available. Several women who describe overcoming infertility with the help of alternative therapists went to them because they had been offered drugs to induce ovulation but were reluctant to take them when they learned of the possible side effects. Several were not told, despite asking the prescribing doctor, and it is undoubtedly true that some fertility drugs are given to women without careful provision having been made for monitoring their response, as recommended by the manufacturers of the drugs.

Disturbing reports are also emerging about the long-term as well as short-term disadvantages of assisted conception. Increased miscarriage levels and premature and multiple births are not only very distressing but have considerable cost implications, both personally and generally. Babies born prematurely, or as one of twins or more, are at a disadvantage from the start, but there are also some reports of increased rates of ovarian cancer in women who have taken fertility drugs and of cancer in the babies of mothers who have had ovulation induced by drugs.

The numbers involved are tiny and doubtless many couples are prepared to take this and many other, more immediate, risks in order to have a baby. They may not, until now, have realized that there were any other paths to pursue. Fortunately, for couples with unexplained infertility—and others—there are alternatives.

A personal view

I am fortunate enough to have several children, most of whom were conceived without difficulty. Therefore, you may not think

I am qualified to write about infertility and it is true that I have no personal experience of primary infertility. Yet, although it may be even less discussed than primary infertility, many couples suffer from secondary infertility, defined as being unable to have the number of children that you want. There is also a subdivision, known technically as infecundity, which is defined as failure to have a live birth and due in my case, and that of many others, not to an inability to become pregnant, but to stay that way until the baby stands a chance of life.

I had recurrent miscarriages for five years and remember, although I would prefer not to, those awful days of despair, rising hope being dashed yet again and a strong feeling that no one had the remotest idea of how I felt. Easy assumptions about being over it, or that it was unimportant, because we already had children, and other such heedless comments or actions went deep. In common with other women who miscarry, especially if it is more than once, I felt it would just about be tolerable if I knew everything would finally be all right, even if it took a long time to happen. It was the uncertainty of our ever succeeding, together with putting life on hold, not starting a new career and always thinking that I could not take on anything very challenging because we might soon have another baby that means I do have some idea of what it is like. Moreover, I was offered inappropriate drugs and investigations and finally told to go home and come to terms with it. I felt no one looked at my case with any real thought or offered any hope.

As a result of our experiences, a colleague and I started a bereavement group for parents who lose babies either during pregnancy or shortly after birth. Quite a few of the people who attended had lost a baby that had taken months or years to conceive. It is a particularly bitter fact that couples who do not conceive easily may experience a higher rate of miscarriage when they do. Yet among those couples are some who have improved their fertility by using alternative therapies. Several of the group members who had had one, two or more miscarriages eventually had the baby they wanted after hearing my story, and consulting a medical herbalist.

Herbal medicine, I felt, was the end of the line for me—I was even reluctant to try it in case it failed. Nothing else had worked. However, three months' treatment together with self-prescribed iron supplements did the trick. Despite fairly hefty stress levels, I became and stayed pregnant and eventually gave birth to a beautiful daughter. Two years later and without any additional treatment, we had a lovely son, born two and a half weeks late at home.

1

THE BACKGROUND TO INFERTILITY

The rate of subfertility is increasing. Current estimates suggest that 15 percent of couples will experience involuntary childlessness during the course of their lives and half that number will not have the number of children that they would like.

This definition encompasses both those who have difficulty in conceiving their first child and those who have already had a child but have problems in achieving pregnancy again. It also includes those who are able to conceive but in whom pregnancy does not result in a live birth, particularly those who miscarry recurrently.

The rate of subfertility is likely to be underestimated, as it includes only those couples who seek medical help for their problem. There are others who are prepared to accept their lack of fertility or who do not conceive, despite having unprotected intercourse, but are not actively trying for a baby. There is some evidence to suggest that couples with secondary infertility are less likely to seek help.[1] Moreover, couples who overcome their fertility problems with the aid of complementary therapies without consulting a doctor may not be included in the statistics for infertility or its successful treatment.

Several factors appear to be responsible for the growing incidence of infertility. First, as public perception of it as a treatable condition grows, people may approach their doctors in order to receive help. The subject is constantly featured in the media and, while it may seem erroneously that every type of fertility problem can be remedied by in vitro fertilization (IVF), recent developments such as intracytoplasmic sperm injection (ICSI)—where a single spem is inserted into an egg via a very fine needle—can certainly offer hope where there was little before.

Secondly, the prevalence of sexually transmitted diseases, such as chlamydia, is growing. There is not enough public awareness that easily acquired and in many cases painless, bacterial infection can be stealthily wrecking women's fallopian tubes and ruining their chances of natural conception, or causing their pregnancies to be ectopic.

Finally, despite reports to the contrary, it is becoming clear that sperm counts are declining generally.

The causes of infertility vary proportionately between those who are experiencing primary infertility and those who are having difficulty following the birth of a child. The graphs below show the relative incidence of the reasons for infertility in these cases.

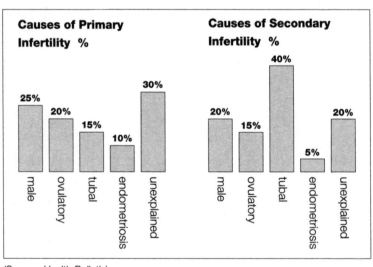

(Source: *Health Bulletin*)

Taken overall, these rates average as follows:

male	25 percent
ovulatory	15 percent
tubal	20 percent
unexplained	25 percent
endometriosis	5 percent

· *Causes of male infertility* ·

It is not yet known what gives sperm the power to fertilize an egg, although a sample can be checked to see whether it is (apparently) normal. It is possible for sperm to appear normal but be unable to fertilize an egg when placed together with eggs during the IVF process. To get a true picture of a man's fertility potential, it is important to have sperm analysed at least two or three times, because there can be substantial variation in sperm counts. According to *The Lancet*, different laboratories use different methods of investigation. This can profoundly affect the diagnosis: one laboratory may rate a man suitable to be a sperm donor while the next describes him as infertile.

There are three possible ways in which sperm may be deficient:

• the number produced
• their ability to propel themselves forward
• the shape of the head

The average sperm count is around 100 million per milliliter, and there may be 3.5 to 13 ml. in an ejaculate. They are produced at a rate of 1,800 per second from each testicle. These seemingly excessive numbers are necessary to fertilize an egg. Counts below 20 to 40 million per milliliter are considered subfertile and those below 20 million per milliliter are considered low (with a poor chance of fertility), although fertilization is not impossible and may just take longer to achieve.

Morphology

Sperm with abnormally shaped heads are generally incapable of fertilization. Humans, unlike animals, often have sperm with abnormalities. According to the World Health Organization (WHO) classification, it can be normal for up to 70 percent of human sperm to be irregularly shaped, including those with heads which are larger or smaller than usual, have narrow heads, have two heads with one tail or two tails with one head.

Motility

Sperm may also have difficulty in moving. The tail of a sperm is designed to thrash about in order to propel itself forward. Some sperm are unable to do this and either move very slowly (normal sperm can reach the fallopian tubes in less than an hour when traveling through favorable mucus), swim erratically in circles or in zigzag patterns, or clump together with other sperm (this is known as agglutination). Obviously, motility is important: there is no value in having a high sperm count if they cannot reach the egg. It is estimated that with a rate of 100 million motile sperm per milliliter there is a 70 percent chance of conceiving; with rates of 5 to 10 million per milliliter, this is reduced to 30 percent.

It is accepted that in general the incidence of disorders of the male reproductive tract is rising, having more than doubled in the last 30 to 50 years,[2] while sperm counts have declined by more than half. Possible reasons for this are discussed on page 94. However, it means that male factor infertility is increasing. Although intracytoplasmic sperm injection (ICSI) has made available a means of treating the symptoms, there is no generally accepted cure for male infertility. In 15 percent of cases no cause can be identified; in the remaining 85 percent a cause can be identified, but it may be descriptive rather than diagnostic. Causes include:

Genetic factors including chromosome abnormalities

Impaired sperm production or function, occurring as a result of:
  genetic reasons
  delayed descent of testes
  mumps
  chlamydia
  cancer
  varicocele (varicose vein in the testes)
  irradiation
  cytotoxic drugs
  other drugs

Environmental agents

Impaired sperm transport due to :
>   auto-immune infertility (where a man produces antibodies
>   in his own sperm)
>   blockage of vas deferens
>   ejaculatory problems

Disturbances in sperm-egg fusion with abnormal egg-binding proteins

Recurrent miscarriage due to chromosomal aberration

Some treatment is available, although it is not always effective and in some cases controversial. For example, some doctors will operate to correct a varicocele, whereas others do not consider this to be helpful. Immunological infertility may be treated successfully with steroids but they can also have serious side effects.[3]

· *Causes of female infertility* ·

Ovulation problems

In normal ovulation and with a cycle lasting 28 days, at the beginning of each cycle follicle-stimulating hormone (FSH) stimulates several follicles (sacs containing eggs) to develop in the ovaries. Granulosa cells around the developing follicles start to grow and to produce estrogen, causing blood levels of estrogen to rise. After about the sixth day one follicle begins to dominate, leaving the others behind. This follicle produces more estrogen, which has the effect of reducing the levels of FSH. As a result, the main follicle continues to grow but the others, unable to survive without FSH, stop growing and regress. The dominant follicle is by then sufficiently mature to survive and continues to grow.

As the follicle matures, a cavity forms around the egg inside it. This fills with fluid, and the egg becomes suspended, attached to a stem. If you were able to see it, this follicle would appear as a bulge on the surface of the ovary, measuring between 2 and 3 centimeters across. Distension of the ovary may result in pain.

At the moment of ovulation, classically at around day 14 of a 28-day cycle, the follicle ruptures and the egg, surrounded by a blob of jelly, bursts forth.

The egg is then wafted to the end of the fallopian tube, which has fingerlike ends surrounding the ovary. Cilia, little hairs within the fallopian tubes, beat to encourage the egg onward down the tube and into the cervix. The now empty follicle collapses and forms the corpus luteum, a yellow cyst which is able to produce the hormones estrogen and progesterone in preparation for pregnancy. If the egg is fertilized and implants, the corpus luteum will continue the hormone production to sustain the pregnancy and prevent a period until the placenta takes over hormone production at thirteen to fourteen weeks, at which time the corpus luteum fades away.

If the egg is not fertilized, it starts to degenerate while still on its five- to seven-day journey down to the uterus. The corpus luteum will continue to produce progesterone until the tenth day after ovulation in a conventional cycle. Then it will stop producing both estrogen and progesterone unless a fertilized egg has implanted in the endometrium, the lining of the uterus. This triggers menstruation and the shedding of the endometrium after a further four days and the release of more FSH and LH from the pituitary gland.

Failure to ovulate may be due to various causes including:

hypergonadotropic hypogonadism
hypothalamic failure
hyperprolactinemia
polycystic ovary syndrome
premature failure of the ovaries
cyst cycles
luteinized unruptured follicle
egg retention
elderly egg
cytotoxic drugs
other drugs
irradiation
smoking

Endometriosis

This disease results in tissue from the endometrium, the lining of the uterus, being found elsewhere in the body, usually in the pelvic cavity. It responds to hormones in the same way as the endometrium, but, as there is no outlet for the blood lost, it tends to form dark brown cysts which may cause adhesions, so that internal organs stick together instead of being able to slide over each other as normal. The resulting symptoms may include heavy periods, painful sex, lower back pain, diarrhea, constipation, and rectal bleeding.

In the past endometriosis was considered to be a considerable cause of infertility, and it is true that where there are adhesions, the anatomy is distorted, or there is ovarian or tubal damage, fertility can be impaired by endometriosis. Formerly women with a diagnosis of endometriosis were urged to become pregnant immediately, no matter how inappropriate this might be for them at the time, partly because pregnancy was thought to be an effective treatment and also because it might prove their only chance of having a baby. However, it is now thought that mild to moderate endometriosis may neither cause infertility nor be cured by pregnancy. It may be that the increase in laparoscopic examinations results in diagnosis of endometriosis being made more frequently when it is not causing problems. It has always been noted that the degree to which endometriosis is apparent may bear little relation to the severity of symptoms. Some women are unaware of having considerable endometriosis until they are examined by laparoscope, while in others little in the way of endometrial plaques can be detected, although they are suffering severe symptoms typical of the condition.

An interesting trial in Spain[4] involved a group of infertile women before they had had a laparoscopy and asked them about their physical symptoms of pelvic pain, painful periods, pain on intercourse, etc. They also examined them physically to see if some of what are considered to be classic signs of endometriosis were present, for example, whether it was painful when they pushed against the cervix, if the uterus was retroverted or not easy to move, whether there were nodules in the uterosacral area or pain without nodules. The doctors then gave each woman the laparoscopy. Somewhat surprisingly, they found that as many women without any evidence of endometriosis (viewed through the laparoscope) had symptoms of the disease as those who did have the disease. Levels of pelvic pain and painful periods were similar: more than half the women in each group had painful periods. There were some differences regarding the presence of uterosacral nodules and pain, which were exclusive to the endometriosis group, but otherwise no significant differences. It seems that discovering that a woman has endometriosis does not necessarily mean that it is the cause of her infertility.

Drug treatment for endometriosis

Endometriosis is commonly treated by giving drugs to suppress ovulation and menstruation, the belief being that, as the endometrial tissue which is within the pelvic cavity but outside the uterus no longer responds to the monthly cycle, the cysts will shrink and disappear. This treatment was given to infertile women with endometriosis in order to restore fertility and may still be prescribed for this reason. It can be useful in reducing symptoms but an overview of 25 randomized controlled trials showed that it was of no significant value in increasing pregnancy rates.[5] The researchers also stated that there was nothing more to be gained by combining drug treatment with conservative surgery (laparotomy), although they considered that laparoscopic surgery using laser treatment looked more promising. However, further work needed to be done in order to be sure.

Drugs taken to suppress ovulation which inhibit pituitary gonadotropins can have serious side effects. They are anti-estrogenic and antiprogesteronic and tend towards a masculinizing effect. Women can be severely affected by taking them and it is important that there be an interval of three months between ceasing to take them and trying to become pregnant as they can cause masculinization of female babies.

The drug danazol and the gonadorelin analogues, used in IVF treatments, can have similar side effects, although the latter are taken by way of a nasal spray (naferelin [Synarel], etc). If they are prescribed for you, you may not be warned about their possible side effects or told when you should avoid taking them.

These drugs should be prescribed with caution if you have any of the following conditions:

Heart, liver or kidney problems
polycythemia
epilepsy
diabetes
high blood pressure
migraines
lipoprotein disorder
a history of thrombosis

They should not be taken in pregnancy so it is important to make sure you are not pregnant (and will not become pregnant) before starting to take them. Neither should they be taken by anyone who has severe forms of any the conditions mentioned above or who has abnormal vaginal bleeding or porphyria.

The side effects include: nausea, dizziness, rashes, backache, mood changes, nervousness, weight gain, menstrual disturbances, flushing, reduction in breast size, skeletal muscle spasm, hair loss, masculinizing effects such as greasy skin, increased body hair growth, swelling and voice deepening (this may not be reversible on stopping the drug), shrinking of the clitoris, leucopenia, thrombocytopenia, intracranial hypertension, visual disturbances, and jaundice.

Tubal damage

Until recently tubal infertility has been treatable only with microsurgery, with a limited amount of success and an increased risk of ectopic pregnancy even when tubes have been cleared.

A new technique of tubal catheterization involving diagnostic X rays, guide wires, and high technology catheters is proving successful in unblocking tubes when the blockage occurs at the end closest to the uterus. If successful, its benefit is that it will allow conception to take place naturally, although there may still be a higher-than-average risk of ectopic pregnancy.

Tubal infertility may be caused by problems present from birth, but in the vast majority it is caused by infection as a result of sexually transmitted diseases which result in pelvic inflammatory disease (PID). Tubal infertility may also be caused by infection following a miscarriage or termination of pregnancy, infection after childbirth, appendicitis when the appendix ruptures, and other forms of peritonitis and abdominal surgery.

Chlamydia

Although not widely known about, *Chlamydia trachomatis,* a bacterial infection, is the most prevalent type of sexually transmitted infection. Occurring in both men and women, it often produces no symptoms, particularly in women, but can climb up through the cervix and into the fallopian tubes, resulting in tissue damage and greatly increasing the chance of ectopic pregnancy or tubal infertility. Each attack of PID increases the likelihood of infertility; more than 10 percent of women who have one attack are rendered infertile, rising to 90 percent with three or more attacks. Three out of four women with tubal infertility or ectopic pregnancy were found to have had chlamydia compared with one in four fertile women.

The infection can take years to develop and is difficult to test for with accuracy. Those who have had the infection longer may be less likely to test positive for it than those who have acquired it in the last six months, although more sensitive tests are being developed.

Symptoms

Seventy percent of women with chlamydia may be unaware that they have it and will find out only when they have problems conceiving, have an ectopic pregnancy or are tested for the disease before a gynecological procedure. Others may have symptoms of vaginal discharge, bleeding between periods, lower abdominal pain, and pain on urination.

In men the infection can cause pain on urination and a discharge, although they too may have no symptoms.

Babies can acquire the disease at birth if their mothers are infected, when it leads to neonatal conjunctivitis and chlamydia pneumonia.

Treatment

Chlamydia and other sexually transmitted diseases are treatable by antibiotics, although if you do not have symptoms, you are unlikely to know that you need treatment. It is estimated that in some areas as many as 12 percent of the population are infected, and it is felt that there should be routine screening for the disease to prevent its serious consequences.

If chlamydia is detected in either partner, both partners must be treated with antibiotics. Doxycycline 100 mg twice daily for seven days is recommended by the Centers for Disease Control, unless a woman is pregnant or breast-feeding, in which case the antibiotic recommended is erythromycin 500 mg four times a day for seven days, or 250 mg four times a day for fourteen days.

If pelvic inflammatory disease is suspected, antichlamydial treatment should last for fourteen days and sex is inadvisable until both partners have completed their treatment. A visit to a gynecological clinic is useful to check that the treatment has been successful and to monitor any other infections.

· *Unexplained infertility* ·

This book is primarily concerned with unexplained infertility, that is infertility where both partners are apparently normal according to all tests. However, it is also relevant to those with other diagnoses for infertility, particularly the descriptive ones (for example, you may have a low sperm count but the reason for it is not known). Figures vary, but as many as 40 percent of cases of infertility have been described as unexplained. Clearly, not enough is yet known about why pregnancy may or may not occur and there is still much to be discovered. Fertilization and implantation and the maintenance of pregnancy are complex processes, affected by many factors, both physical and emotional.

It may be tempting to regard infertility as purely physical—a belief that tends to be endorsed by the medical profession, who will treat the problem symptomatically, even in the absence of a diagnosis (as with IUI or superovulation—see page 53). However, this approach often overlooks the ways in which couples may be able to overcome their problems by taking responsibility for themselves, rather than handing it over to the doctors.

It can be hard to accept that the answer may lie in your own hands, just as it can be unsatisfactory for a doctor to recommend changes in lifestyle rather than handing over a prescription. As with medical treatment, although there are no guarantees, there is growing evidence that steps you can take yourselves, together with the help you may seek from practitioners of alternative therapies, can make the difference between unexplained infertility and pregnancy. For example, underweight women who rarely have a period and do not ovulate can become pregnant naturally after gaining weight, when they generally start to menstruate normally. Equally, overweight women with polycystic ovaries have found themselves able to conceive after losing weight. Many of the women who tell their stories in this book have conceived after years of infertility following visits to a reflexologist or healer.

Although other women may seem to become pregnant with no difficulty at all, and even when they don't want to, human reproduction is notoriously inefficient, and for many people being only slightly off-balance physiologically may be sufficient to prevent conception. Each couple is different; only those trying to become pregnant will really know how they are affected by infertility, or have a good idea about what might help, or know exactly how motivated either partner is to make beneficial changes. It may appear that making changes will involve a huge upheaval. A man with a low sperm count who spends all day at the wheel will probably find it hard to change or give up his job, particularly if he is not able to do anything else (see pages 100–101). It will be even harder if he, or his partner, are not convinced that this will make a difference.

It can also be very hard to accept that you may subconsciously be holding back from parenthood. However, it is clear from talking to people with fertility problems and the practitioners who treat them that it is quite possible for mental blocks to prevent pregnancy taking place. You may be unaware of reasons that make you reluctant to become pregnant; and it is not easy to believe that events in your past can have such a powerful physical effect. However, the fact that women who have undergone long periods of infertility have been successfully treated by hypnotherapy means that infertility can be caused by emotional as well as physical reasons.

Stress, too, can cause problems. The question of whether stress can lead to infertility or vice versa has been researched and debated at length. There is little doubt, though, that infertility is stressful. There certainly are women who reflect stress by changes in their menstrual cycle, often quite dramatically. It is quite possible that humans, like other animals, put on physiological brakes while they are under stress, because their bodies decide that it is not a good time for conception. Men, too, can show a reaction to stress, by a fall in their sperm count; in fact, counts often decline just before a sample is required to be produced for IVF treatment, despite having been at normal levels until then.

THE EMOTIONAL EFFECTS

When subfertile couples start trying to have a baby, they are in most instances just the same as other couples. They are likely to have used contraception, in the belief that they are fertile, and will have made plans in the expectation of becoming parents. They may even have chosen each other partly on the basis of the sort of father or mother they think their partner is likely to be.

Only as time goes by will they begin to wonder whether there is a problem, a doubt that becomes reinforced as their contemporaries seem to conceive easily. How long couples wait before agreeing to consult a doctor or other practitioner will depend on their personalities, their degree of optimism, their faith in medicine, their sense of their ability to affect their lives, and on other factors, including their ages. They are unlikely to want to focus on having a baby if they are experiencing marital instability, if they are in financial difficulty, or if family members are ill.

Talking to someone else about subfertility can be a big step. Consulting a doctor about any medical problem can increase your anxiety, and describing your difficulties in conceiving can be particularly daunting. This is not only because it is an area where you may not be sure of the response—you may be worried that your GP will say you have not been trying for long enough (and many doctors will not refer you to a specialist unless you have been trying to conceive for over a year)—but also because it is an intensely private problem which people are reluctant to talk about, and of which they fear the outcome.

It is difficult for other people to realize how unhappy failing to conceive may make couples feel. They may tend to put off seeking help for fear of receiving a clear-cut diagnosis of infertility. People who are afraid they may have cancer often make a similar delay: they feel that they can remain hopeful if no one confirms the dreaded diagnosis.[1] Making an appointment to discuss fertility sometimes seems tantamount to handing over control, and loss of control is one of the aspects of infertility that couples dislike most. For many it may be the first time in their lives that they have encountered anything which cannot be overcome by hard work. It can be embarrassing and humiliating to discuss your intimate sexual behavior with a third party, especially when the reason for attending makes you feel diminished and less of a man or woman. It is normal for couples to feel anxious, angry and guilty, particularly if they think that their past behavior is responsible for their current difficulties. It is common for people with fertility problems to have low self-esteem, to be irritable, to become introverted, and to feel neurotic and isolated from the rest of the world.

Couples may wait a long time before starting to view themselves as having a problem with fertility. Each month brings its own cycle of hope and despair and with it feelings of shock, dismay, loss of control, and difficulty in accepting that pregnancy is not occurring as planned. Partly because it is reasonable not to expect to become pregnant immediately and also because you are unlikely to be offered medical help unless you have been trying for six to twelve months, you may be able to justify not seeking treatment while the realization that things are not going according to plan slowly dawns on you. There is always the hope that it might happen next month and couples may be reluctant to involve a third party, who may not treat them sympathetically, and so at this stage they may not admit to themselves that they have a problem.[2]

You may find it even harder to come to terms with infertility if you experience it once you have already had a child. It can be very difficult to believe that you cannot become pregnant again if you found it easy to conceive before. You will actually know what you are missing and feel the loss of a real child rather than the fantasy baby that you imagine before you have had a baby. You are likely to be surrounded by women who are becoming pregnant without difficulty, and may tell yourself that you ought to be grateful for what you have, while still wanting another.

A GP may well recognize and understand these feelings and realize that anyone who has taken the step of asking for help wants it at the time they ask for it, and does not what to be told to allow nature to take its course. However, the medical viewpoint may differ from yours, because, although the majority of couples conceive within a few months, for a minority it will take longer and spontaneous pregnancies do occur even after twelve months of trying. Indeed, 18 percent of couples in one survey who had been on an IVF program and failed to conceive, having had fertility problems for more than five years, did not return for embryo transfer because they had conceived spontaneously subsequently.[3] One expert[4] recommends four years of trying before using assisted conception methods.

Couples may find it hard to talk to a doctor, but they can also find it hard to talk to each other. They may feel acute pain and anxiety individually but try to protect their partner by not admitting to it. Embarking on tests which may reveal that one of them is responsible for the "failure" to procreate, is nerve-racking. When either the man or the woman has a fertility problem, they may find it hard to believe at first. The partner diagnosed as normal may feel angry at the other, and guilt about previous lifestyle, partners, abortions, pelvic infections, etc. can also increase anger and feelings of defectiveness. Anger may be expressed at health professionals and it is important at this point and throughout that people are given accurate information and that knowledge is shared with them.

The partner with the fertility problem will not only feel guilty and that it is all his or her fault, but may also fear that the other person will leave the relationship for someone with whom they can have a baby. The fertile partner may indeed fantasize about leaving—partly to escape the anguish and partly to have a chance of having a baby. Couples may find themselves either driven apart or united. They may feel punished and question whether they should even be married if they cannot produce a child. Some religions are particularly hard on infertile couples, although there has been a recent breakthrough in the Catholic Church, which stated that it has no moral or ethical objections to a new tubal catheterization procedure to unblock fallopian tubes. Hitherto Catholic couples have been barred by their religion from having IVF treatment.[5]

Grief follows anger; infertility has been described as "chronic sorrow."[6] It represents a potential loss rather than an actual one and it is even harder to talk about than bereavement. Many people find that other people cannot deal sensitively with the loss of a baby at miscarriage, still less with the feelings of distress at failing to become pregnant. Moreover, because there is still always hope, each month brings the possibility that the grief may be resolved by pregnancy, unlike in bereavement, where there is no possibility of resolving the sadness other than by coming to accept it. This distressing state can often put people, women in particular, into a state of limbo where they cannot put their sad experiences behind them and move on, because they may become pregnant at any time. This can have particular bearing on careers: women may not want to change direction or job if they feel they will not continue with it should they become pregnant. It is a very uncertain time and it may be difficult to feel as though you have any control over the situation. Seeking medical treatment can be seen as useful, because it focuses on the problem and offers the means to do something about it, while at the same time it is something to which people submit—it is done to them or for them and they rarely feel that it is under their control.

Medical treatment has disadvantages in its own right: it can be painful or cause other health problems, it may not be administered sympathetically or sensitively and when paid for privately can be frighteningly expensive. Accommodating tests and treatment can be difficult when they interfere with work, especially if you don't want to discuss the reason for taking time off, or if your employers are unsympathetic.

The couple may also be out of synchrony, one may want to go ahead with treatment, while the other has not yet come to terms with a test result or is reluctant to take that particular step. Unless both partners are allowed time to consider their feelings, they may find themselves pressured into a hasty ill-judged decision that they may later regret.

In addition, it may seem difficult—even impossible—to talk about infertility problems with your family or friends. Society does not understand the feelings of infertile couples and people find it hard to know what to say or do to support them. In their desire to make things better, they often say things that appear very insensitive. Even couples in this situation concede that it is hard to say the right thing and that, depending on their mood, they may welcome or reject the same remark. Some people do show a lack of empathy or imagination, however, and anyone who wants to make infertile couples feel better would be well advised to steer clear of any comment that starts "At least . . . ." (as in "At least you can have fun trying"). Other remarks, including "Just relax," "Why don't you get a kitten?" and "You wouldn't really want children anyway," can cause deep hurt and frustration. Even if you do have a friend in whom you find it easy to confide, you may worry that they will become bored with your continuing difficulties.

If people are aware of your problems it can lead to awkward social situations. You may be the last to hear of a pregnancy because no one wants to upset you; other people may feel constrained in your presence and unable to talk freely about pregnancy, babies or children; you may wish to avoid situations where you know that children, especially those of your brother or sister may be present, thus increasing your sense of isolation.

It is no wonder that many couples become quite secretive about their problems, realizing that if they don't admit to their difficulties no one will be able to make hurtful comments about them. Unfortunately, if infertility is not discussed openly by those who are suffering from it, it will remain a taboo subject and society will continue to be unaware of the feelings of infertile couples.

Moreover, although the state of infertility has been likened to mourning for a child that has not existed, unlike mourning a death, there is no point until the menopause at which it can be said that there is definitely no hope. Each month, hopes may be raised particularly when a period is late, symptoms examined minutely and perhaps early pregnancy tests bought, only for all hope to be dashed disastrously with the start of bleeding. The grief and depression can be intense, fading as the next opportunity for conception approaches. Meanwhile, it can feel as though life is permanently on hold, being careful about diet and alcohol and avoiding smoking, seemingly to no avail.

There is no ritual to recognize and overcome this frequent loss, just as there is still no recognized grieving ritual for babies who start to develop and then die during pregnancy. Miscarriage, like infertility, is a subject that is frequently unappreciated and unrecognized, except by the parents and those who have had a similar experience. The intensity of grief can leave women in particular, feeling as though they are going mad and suffering even more because such emotions are not generally known to be normal.

Women do bear the brunt of the emotional and physical distress of childlessness. They are ten times more likely to initiate a consultation about the problem and the majority of tests, particularly those which are most intrusive or painful, such as the hysterosalpingogram, hysteroscopy or laparoscopy, are performed on women. Investigations and treatment are likely to be more time-consuming and arduous for the woman and the risks to her health will be proportionately greater. Women are much more likely to become depressed and anxious about it all (30 percent, as opposed to 18 percent of men), not least because child-bearing is seen as so much more important for women. Girls are brought up to expect to become mothers, it is much more central to their upbringing than the prospect of fatherhood is to a boy's. Men tend to find it easier than women to sublimate their desire for parenthood into working hard at their job, although a woman may be able to discuss her problems more readily and seek help more easily. For her it is much more difficult to suppress the strong biological desire for a child.

Some women and couples may become so driven by their longing for a baby that they are able to think of little else and the quality of the rest of their lives declines unnecessarily dramatically. It is easy to sympathize with such people, who will take any opportunity, however remote. In one study, 20 percent of women and 7 percent of men said that they would give up everything in order to have a baby.[7] Another study showed that 50 percent of couples were still going for medical treatment after six years and that 93 percent of women who had recently had a failed attempt at IVF would try anything new. Couples were described as having "tunnel vision," ready to try any treatment, even if it had a very low success rate.[8, 9]

In this situation it is possible to become dependent on the doctors treating you, feeling that they are the only ones that understand or offer any hope; but you may lose your critical ability to assess what they are offering in terms of value, possible success, and risks to yourselves. You may feel that you have to be "good patients" and suspend any objective criticism that you otherwise might make. It can be difficult to get past this, to realize that there may be alternatives and view the situation objectively, rather than seeing only as far as the next medically-assisted attempt at conception.

Men, although statistically less affected emotionally than women, do find the process very taxing. Many feel very angry about the situation and the ways in which they are treated by doctors. They complain about the insensitive ways in which they are told about their problem, and about their situation being discussed with their partners but not with them. They say that their feelings are not addressed in the fertility programs and that provision made for them is poor or nonexistent, insensitive and frequently degrading. Their male friends and colleagues may be very unkind, joking about masculinity and sexual prowess. Men in the armed services can find it particularly hard to cope with infertility treatment.[10]

The stage of grief or sorrow may reach an end when the couple have a child (either naturally, by using assisted conception or egg or sperm donation, or through adoption), when the grief is resolved, or when the partnership breaks down. When infertility results in a baby, the grief is over, although the legacy of infertility may continue to cause problems in pregnancy and thereafter (see Chapter 7). However, when infertility continues, as we have seen, there may be no definite end unless couples define one for themselves or menopause puts their hopes beyond reach. That particular difficulty is now compounded by the advent of the new assisted reproductive techniques (ARTs) which can prolong the process. Methods that offer new hope are to be welcomed, but they may mean that people's lives remain in limbo for longer and they are not able to move on. When ICSI first became available, offering men with very low sperm count a chance of fatherhood, the technique was offered to couples who had come to feel that they must accept their childlessness.[11] When the clinic wrote to them offering the procedure, some saw it as a wonderful opportunity while others regarded it as reopening old wounds and resented it. Many will only come to terms with infertility when the biological clock stops ticking; they cannot move through the stages of grief—denial, anger, and acceptance—while hope remains.

However, as this book shows, there are ways of improving your quality of life, maximizing opportunities, promoting relaxation and improving health which, even if they do not result in the birth of a baby, will increase your ability to enjoy life while you continue to try to overcome your difficulties.

•

3

MEDICAL AND
SURGICAL FERTILITY
TREATMENTS

It is evident that men and women are not well informed about the drawbacks to fertility treatments, even when they specifically ask about them. Some risks are high—for example, the chance of having a multiple birth if you take gonadotropins—and some are extremely low, such as the concern that babies of mothers who have taken ovulation-inducing drugs will develop cancer in infancy. Other effects of fertility treatment, such as the future impact on the fertility of babies born as a result of ICSI treatment, are speculative or unknown. The disadvantages may not be limited to medical treatments; the lack of research into alternative treatments for infertility means there may be drawbacks to them too. However, they work largely by helping the body to function better rather than forcing it work. For example, the treatment might help the pituitary gland work correctly in conjunction with the rest of the body, rather than being kicked into action with drugs while other factors are missing or not coordinated.

· *Drugs* ·

It is useful to look at fertility drugs and their effects because it is clear that some are prescribed for longer than the manufacturers recommend, and women's responses to the drugs in particular are not always adequately monitored. Let's begin with the most frequently prescribed fertility drugs.

Clomid/serophene, clomiphene citrate

How it works

Clomid was first synthesized in 1956 and first used in chemical trials in 1960. It is thought to react with estrogen-receptors in the hypothalamus to suppress natural estrogen levels. This encourages the body to produce more gonadotropins, which stimulates follicles of the ovaries to grow and increases the production of luteinizing hormones which enable them to develop. It is also useful in the subsequent development of the corpus luteum.

Who should be given it

Clomid should be prescribed for women who fail to ovulate, ovulate only rarely, or have a history of limited ovulation. It is sometimes used for those with luteal phase defects (where the endometrium does not prepare to receive an egg in synchrony with its release from the ovary). This drug was formerly used in IVF treatment, but was later thought to result in reduced fertility and recurrent miscarriage.

Clomid can promote more frequent ovulation and helps to time ovulation more accurately, which is useful when artificial insemination is performed. It is suitable for women with good levels of endogenous estrogen, as evidenced by vaginal smears, endometrial biopsy, urinary estrogen, and endometrial bleeding in response to progesterone.

Who should not be given it

- Anyone who has had a deep vein thrombosis[1]
- Women who are ovulating
- Women who have low-weight amenorrhea
- Women with primary pituitary or ovarian failure
- Women with ovulatory failure due to thyroid or adrenal disorders
- Women with hyperprolactinemia
- Women with high FSH levels due to early menopause
- Anyone with ovarian cysts
- Anyone with liver disease or dysfunction

Precautions

Clomid should be taken only when a pelvic examination to exclude the possibility of ovarian cysts has been carried out, at the start of each course of treatment. It should be prescribed for women with polycystic ovaries only with caution.

The recommended dose

Women should take one 50 mg tablet daily for five days, starting on the fifth day of the cycle, that is, from the fifth to the ninth day. If ovulation occurs, the dosage should be maintained at this level. The majority of women who are going to respond to Clomid will do so with the first course. Three cycles should be sufficient. Intercourse must be timed to coincide with ovulation.

If ovulation does not occur, the dosage can be increased to 100 mg daily for five days, but no higher dose should be prescribed. It is recommended that it be prescribed for three cycles only.

Short-term side effects

- Ovarian enlargement (in 13.6 percent of women)
- Hot flashes (in 10.4 percent of women)
- Abdominal or pelvic discomfort—bloating or distension. This occurs in around 5 percent of women and should be reported immediately. It may take several days to subside once the drug is stopped.
- Eye symptoms, such as blurred vision or seeing spots or flashes. If you have these symptoms you should stop taking the drug immediately.
- Skin rashes and nettle rash.
- Rarely (in fewer than 1 percent of women): dizziness, lightheadedness, giddiness, nervous tension, insomnia, fatigue, and depression.
- Cervical mucus abnormalities. Clomid can reduce production of the thin mucus of ovulation that is essential for fertilization although the high levels of estrogen produced by multiple follicles developing may correct the balance. This occurs in up to 59 percent of cases.

• Luteinized unruptured follicle syndrome. This is associated with Clomid, but is not necessarily more common than in other infertile women. It happens when ovulation occurs but the egg is not released and the follicle collapses.[2]

Other effects

There is a higher than average rate of miscarriage with Clomid. This may be due to several reasons, including the defects it can cause in the luteal phase if given to women who are ovulating, the effect the drug has on cervical mucus and the endometrium, and the higher level of chromosomally abnormal eggs induced by taking Clomid. One study took 177 women who were taking Clomid and recorded their fertilization rates by means of very sensitive tests that measured Early Pregnancy Factor, systemic molecules which are released when the egg and sperm fuse, but before implantation has taken place. It was found that around 80 percent of fertilized eggs failed to implant or develop, although just under half of the women had eggs which were fertilized. Of course there is no way on knowing how frequently this occurs with natural ovulation.[3] Moreover, early pregnancy loss after being on Clomid is often a positive predictor of normal pregnancy in the future.

Multiple gestation

Clomid stimulates a rise in circulating levels of pituitary gonadotropins which results in multiple ovarian follicles. Multiple ovulation increases the numbers of fraternal twins or higher order multiples (up to sextuplets); the vast majority are twins. One large study of 2,369 women who became pregnant while taking Clomid found that

92.1 percent had single babies (2182)
6.9 percent had twins (163)
0.5 percent had triplets (11)
0.13 percent had quadruplets (3)
0.13 percent had quintuplets (3)

Long-term effects on mother and baby

Concern has been expressed about the possibility that taking fertility drugs, including Clomid, can increase the chances of a women developing ovarian cancer.[4] This serious form of cancer affects one woman in eighty in the United States. Several studies, in an effort to determine whether the likelihood of contracting it is increased by taking Clomid, have found that its incidence is greater in infertile women. Whether or not this is because the factor responsible for infertility predisposes a women to ovarian cancer is not yet clear. Some studies have found a higher incidence (nearly three times as great) among infertile women who have taken Clomid than that among infertile women who have not taken Clomid. Other studies have not shown this link and as yet there is no evidence for a cause-and-effect relationship.

However, even those studies which were inconclusive recommend that doctors bear in mind the possible link and be vigilant in monitoring for ovarian cancer. One of the problems is that it may not produce any clear-cut symptoms until it is widespread. Often the only indications are vague abdominal discomfort and swelling. There may also be digestive problems, like nausea and vomiting, together with abnormal vaginal bleeding and excess fluid in the abdominal cavity. It may be possible to feel a swelling in the pelvis. It is clearly important to have any such symptoms checked, whether you have taken fertility drugs or not.

On the plus side, it looks as though Clomid may reduce the chances of getting cervical cancer and there may also be a reduction in the incidence of breast cancer among women who have taken the drug.[5]

Risks to the baby

Concern has also been raised about the probability of long-term effects on the babies of mothers who have taken drugs to induce ovulation.[6] One source [7] quotes several reports that refer to the possibility of Clomid causing neural tube defects, such as anencephaly and spina bifida, in babies. The evidence is not conclusive, but the studies vary between finding no increase in such defects as a result of Clomid, and finding a six-fold increase. Further research of a prospective nature, that is, following mothers taking Clomid through to delivery, rather than asking them later about what drugs they took, may provide a conclusive answer.

Doctors in Australia and Japan have also voiced worries that clomiphene taken by mothers can result in a higher-than-average-level of malignant tumors in their children.[8] Clomid has been safely taken by millions of women around the world and is most unlikely to give a child cancer. However, it has been hypothesized that some drugs, including clomiphene, can induce tumor growth in rodents.[9] Its analogue tamoxifen, sometimes used in fertility treatment for its antiestrogenic effect, has been shown to increase the incidence of uterine and gastrointestinal cancer and to accelerate the growth of gastric cancer, and it is believed that the lowest doses may be the most toxic.

Neuroblastoma is a tumor of the adrenal glands, most develop in the glands or along the back wall of the abdomen. It usually develops within the first four years of life and the incidence is 8.3 cases per million children. Symptoms include weight loss, aches and pains, paleness, and irritability. Some are relatively harmless but others may be very malignant. A recent study[10] suggests that there is a significant increase in the incidence of neuroblastoma in the children of mothers who used fertility drugs, but that taking vitamin supplements in pregnancy seems to have a protective effect.

Possibly an intake of folic acid and vitamins by mothers taking Clomid would protect their babies from the small risk of developing a neural tube defect or neuroblastoma.

Gonadotropins

These are used for women who fail to conceive or ovulate on clomiphene. They may also be used to hyperstimulate the ovaries of women undergoing assisted reproductive techniques such as IVF. The drugs consist of human menopausal gonadotropins, or hMG (obtained from convents) and consist of combined luteinizing hormone and follicle-stimulating hormone (FSH). They are administered once or twice a day by intramuscular injection from day five of the menstrual cycle and should be monitored by the use of ultrasound to gauge the response of the ovaries to the drug. They should not be given to anyone with an ovarian cyst or who is already pregnant or ovulating naturally.

Blood tests are also done to check serum estradiol levels. When they reach 300 pg/ml and one or more follicles has reached a mature size of 18 mm or more, 5,000 to 10,000 IU of human chorionic gonadotropin (hCG) is injected. This should initiate ovulation between 34 and 36 hours later.

The cycle may be abandoned (i.e., hCG not given or intercourse recommended against) if more than three mature follicles develop, if estradiol levels are higher than 2000 pg/ml, or if it looks as though the ovaries have been overstimulated. Extra doses of hCG may be given.

Short-term side effects

About 5 percent of women fail to respond and 5 to 10 percent have to have their cycle canceled because they produce more than three follicles. Early miscarriages occur in 16 to 24 percent of pregnancies conceived in this way.

Intramuscular injections can lead to local irritation at the injection site, or signs of hypersensitivity, such as fever, chills, muscle pains and generally feeling unwell. The large increase in estrogen levels following the stimulation of multiple follicles can also cause nausea, vomiting, diarrhea, abdominal bloating and breast tenderness and discomfort.

Long-term and serious side effects

The risk of developing ovarian cancer after taking gonadotropins is similar to that of taking Clomid. Ovarian hyperstimulation syndrome (OHSS) is a potentially life-threatening side effect of taking fertility drugs, particularly gonadotropins. It is caused by the ovary producing large numbers of follicles in response to the drugs given, rather than just one or two. The numbers can be much greater—as many as 80 and even if the lutenizing hormone drug is not given, the side effects can be alarming. There are degrees of the syndrome, ranging from abdominal pain and marked ovarian enlargment in the less severe cases (these symptoms occur in 3 to 5 percent of women undergoing treatment) to the severe form, which affects between 2 and 23.3 percent of women. [11]

Severe OHSS results in fluid from the follicles collecting in the abdomen. Large amounts of fluid can be involved: as much as 65 liters has been recorded.[12] This leads to weight gain, difficulty in breathing, a fall in blood pressure, fluid in the lungs, and an abdomen severely swollen by all the fluid it contains. The woman also becomes dehydrated and may have problems with her electrolyte balance. Her blood will be more concentrated and so liable to clot too readily. There is a risk of thromboembolism and heart failure.

Her ovaries too will be at risk, having grown to as much as 8 to 10 cm. They will be friable and at risk of rupture, so that any examination should be by gentle ultrasound alone (no pelvic or abdominal examinations). It is possible for the ovaries to rupture, and they may, very rarely, have to be removed to control hemorrhage.[13]

The following women are considered to be at particular risk of developing OHSS.

- Women who are younger than 35
- Women who are lean (underweight)
- Women who have an excessively high estradiol response on the day of hCG administration (4000– 6000 pg/ml)
- Women who have more than 35 follicles yielding more than 30 eggs (considered by some authorities to increase the likelihood of getting OHSS to 80 percent)[14]

Multiple gestation

Perhaps not surprisingly, the chance of a multiple pregnancy is greatly increased by taking gonadotropins. The overall risk is assessed as being nearly 30 percent.[15] One-third of these multiple pregnancies are triplets or more. Of 106 sets of triplets treated in an Israeli hospital:

    7 percent were "natural" (conceived without fertility treatment)
    15 percent resulted from Clomid treatment
    53 percent were conceived after use of gonadotropins
    25 percent were born as a result of IVF

Although the idea of having more than one baby may be appealing, there can be serious threats to the health of multiple babies and their chances of survival. Twins or triplets will make very heavy demands on your time, energy, and finances, and the amount of time you will have to enjoy each baby will be diminished.

The babies are much more likely to be born or delivered prematurely, and there is an increased likelihood of having them by cesarean section. This may follow a pregnancy which will not only have been extra uncomfortable, but may have involved periods of hospitalization for rest, raised blood pressure, anemia or other complications less common among women pregnant with one baby. The babies may also be of low birth-weight, commonly held to be a predisposing factor for ill health in later life. Babies that are small or very small for their gestational age are at increased risk of having heart disease, diabetes, lung disease, and being obese as adults.

There is also the probability that triplets and, to a lesser extent, twins may require intensive resuscitation at birth and have to spend long periods of time in a neonatal special care unit in order to survive. Having children in a special care unit can be extremely taxing and draining even when all goes well, but babies who are born weighing very little or who are born many weeks before they are due, run a greater risk of being damaged or not surviving. It is said that the chances of a baby having cerebral palsy are 8 times higher for twins and 47 times higher for triplets,[16] and it is estimated that twin or triplet survivors may be as much as three times as likely as a single baby to have a severe handicap.[17]

If you want to find out more about life with twins, triplets or more, contact the National Organization of Mothers of Twins Club (see Useful Addresses). They will be able to put you in touch with parents of multiples and can provide support and advice if you find that you are expecting more than one baby.

Bromocriptine

Prolactin is the hormone produced by the pituitary gland which is associated with milk production following pregnancy. It can also suppress ovulation and menstruation during breast-feeding. Some women (as many as one in seven without periods) who have neither been pregnant nor have breast-fed also have high levels of this hormone, which prevents them from menstruating or ovulating. The condition, hyperprolactinemia, which may be associated with stress, can be treated with bromocriptine. This drug acts on the pituitary gland to suppress production of prolactin and allow ovulation to take place. It is effective in restoring ovulation and periods in 95 percent of cases and pregnancy occurs within six months in 35 to 75 percent of women treated with it.

It should only be taken by women with proven hyperprolactinemia on blood testing and should be stopped as soon as conception is confirmed. No more than 1.25 mg per day should be taken for the first week; the dose can then be gradually increased in 1.26-mg increments.

Side effects

Bromocriptine seems to be safe in the long term but has short-term side effects which can be sufficiently severe to cause 5 percent of women to stop taking it.[18] These may include nausea, vomiting, headaches, nasal stuffiness and abdominal cramps. Dizziness on standing is also common, but it is likely to disappear as treatment continues. Other possible side effects are alcohol intolerance, bleeding into the stomach, painful fingers and toes in cold weather, and confusion.

Gonadotropin-releasing hormone pulsatile pump (Pulsatile GnRH)

This treatment is used to mimic the body's own production of luteinizing hormone and FSH. It is suitable only for women with a functional pituitary gland and ovary, unlike gonadotropins, which only require a functional ovary. As it produces results closer to a natural ovulatory cycle, there are fewer of the risks of ovarian stimulation and multiple pregnancies that are associated with gonadotropins. This treatment does not require a further drug to stimulate ovulation and when given to the right people (i.e. those with anovulation due to a shortage of natural gonadotropins and estrogen), it can result in ovulation rates of up to 100 percent.[19]

The disadvantage is that the body naturally produces surges of these hormones approximately every 90 minutes, and in order to produce a similar effect the drug has to be administered by means of a pump and via a needle into a vein or under the skin.

Pregnancy rates are 27 percent per cycle, except for women with polycystic ovaries, for whom it is 13 percent. In this group, pre-treatment with a GnRH agonist proved helpful, pregnancy rates being 71 percent with pre-treatment, as opposed to 49 percent without.[20]

Side effects

Pulsatile GnRH has fewer side effects than other forms of ovulation induction because it is closer to the normal cycle. However, there are obvious disadvantages to having to wear an intravenous pump all the time and there can be problems with the skin, risking inflammation of the vein and clot formation. The needle can easily become displaced and need repositioning. OHSS is rare with pulsatile GnRH but may be developed by women with polycystic ovaries or those who are given excessively high doses of the drug. Multiple pregnancy is less common, occurring in only 8.3 percent of women treated. In most cases only one follicle develops.

Other side effects include headache, nausea, light-headedness, abdominal discomfort, and hot flashes.

· *In Vitro Fertilization (IVF)* ·

Offered as the answer to every infertile couple's problems, IVF is a costly procedure, both financially and emotionally and also in terms of time, health, and its comparatively low success rate.

Many people are not aware of the amount of testing that is required before undergoing IVF, or the frequency with which drugs need to be taken and how they can affect the body. The drugs may either not work at all or work too well, so that the cycle has to be abandoned. An abandoned cycle is not uncommon, despite all the time, effort, and discomfort involved in reaching that stage. A book which gives a fuller idea of what is involved and is well worth reading if you are contemplating assisted conception is Sally Keble's *Conceiving your Baby—How Medicine Can Help* (see Further Reading).

In the UK, IVF and allied procedures such as GIFT (Gamete intrafallopian transfer) and superovulation with IUI (intrauterine insemination), collectively known as ARTs (assisted reproductive techniques), are well regulated, and clinics that provide these services have to be registered and are required to publish their results. Moreover, they are not allowed to put more than three embryos into a woman. In the United States, regulation is voluntary and statistics about success rates less subject to external audit. Unenforceable regulations appear to lead to extensive duplicated tests with overuse of laparoscopy, hysteroscopy, and procedures with a low success rate: treatment such as clomiphene may be used for longer than is reasonable (for example, for nine to twelve months), between three and six embryos may be transferred at one time—sometimes even more.[21] The costs are phenomenal: even before paying the physician's charges or for having the ART, it is estimated that the cost of a single baby is nearly $10,000, while triplets will cost almost $37,000. Sixty to eighty percent of multiple births in the United States are due to ART.

Dr. M. Yusoff Dawood comments[22] that in recent times it would be almost unheard of to unleash drugs or devices into medicine without long and exhaustive research evaluations, yet many new techniques, including some used in assisted conception, are adopted clinically before such assessments are completed.

Although you may understandably be eager to try what

might seem like the only hope of having a baby, it is important to consider the effect that assisted conception may have on the health of the mother and her potential babies. The couples who undergo this process should be those for whom it is the only opportunity to have a child. There is a background rate of spontaneous pregnancy among couples awaiting IVF, and even among those in whom it has failed, and two studies have demonstrated a conception rate leading to live birth of 14.3 to 16.9 percent annually in infertile couples who were not currently receiving any treatment for their failure to conceive.[23] These figures are worth noting when considering whether to embark on expensive and invasive procedures. Several authorities consider that with unexplained infertility a cumulative pregnancy rate of 40 to 65 percent will be achieved within three years.[24]

If a woman has no fallopian tubes, IVF is the only answer, but evidently there are a number of couples who believed that IVF was their only chance of having a baby but conceived naturally either before using the technique or after they had tried it unsuccessfully.

How it works

The woman is given gonadotropin inhibiting drugs (for example, naferelin [Synarel]) to suppress her natural cycle and put her into an artificial and temporary menopause, so that there is no chance of her naturally produced hormones interfering with the carefully synchronized IVF program. This is known as down-regulation and is likely to involve using a nasal spray several times a day, although the drug may also be taken as a subcutaneous injection once a day. The course may last for only a few days or for as long as four weeks. The effects that it has on a woman are similar to those associated with menopause.

The next step is the administration of hMG (human menopausal gonadotropin, see page 41), which is given as an intramuscular injection into the buttock. This stimulates several follicles to develop rather than one, as would occur naturally, and the woman should be carefully monitored under ultrasound. She may need to continue with the nasal spray or subcutaneous injections at the same time.

When the follicles are judged to be of the right size and maturity, she is given an injection of hCG (see page 42) to mimic the surge in luteinizing hormone which normally triggers ovulation. Thirty-five hours later, the eggs are collected, either by laparoscopy or via the vagina, before the follicles rupture spontaneously and the eggs begin to migrate down the fallopian tube. The operation is carried out under general anesthetic or possibly vaginally under sedation alone.

At the same time that the eggs are collected, the male partner has to provide a semen sample which is then treated centrifugally or via liquid to prepare it to be used in fertilization.

The eggs and sperm are placed together in a special culture in a petri dish, by an embryologist. If successful, fertilization will take place within the next 24 to 48 hours. Then the embryos that appear to be of the best quality are transferred directly into the woman's uterus via a catheter, where it is hoped they will implant into the endometrium. Natural implantation takes between five and seven days from fertilization, so that with IVF the embryos arrive in the uterus earlier than they would naturally. Some clinics will administer progesterone in order to increase the likelihood of pregnancy, although this is still debated among many doctors.

There is then a two-week wait to discover whether the eggs have implanted and the woman is pregnant. Unfortunately, hormone levels caused by the drugs can make a woman feel pregnant even when she is not, so that the arrival of a period following IVF treatment can be particularly devastating.

Who should have IVF

It is suitable for women with fallopian tubes that are missing, damaged or blocked beyond doubt on both sides. It is also appropriate for those who have undergone a premature menopause, who have ovaries that cannot be made to ovulate, and in some cases when sperm or eggs are donated.

Who should not have it

Couples who have been trying to conceive for less than a year with intact fallopian tubes in the woman.

Short-term side effects

Human chorionic gonadotropin (hCG) occurs naturally and is obtained from the urine of pregnant women. The injection is likely to be painful—side effects include headache, fatigue, and mood changes.

The down-regulating drugs used in IVF and also to treat endometriosis, such as naferelin, have the effect of inducing artificial menopause and so can have side effects similar to menopausal symptoms. These include breakthrough bleeding, hot flashes, increased sweating, vaginal dryness, changes in libido, headache, nausea, mood changes including depression, changes in breast size, breast tenderness, abdominal pain, fatigue, weight changes, nervousness, dizziness, drowsiness, acne, dry skin, back pain, ovarian cysts (the drug may have to be withdrawn if these develop), decrease in bone density, nettle rash, rash, pruritus vulvae (itchy vulva), constipation, vomiting, sleep disorders, leukorrhea, palpitations, sensitivity of extremities, changes in body hair, and irritation of the inside of the nose.

Long-term side effects

The drawbacks include the risks of multiple births and the risks associated with taking the drugs. There is also a higher incidence of premature labor and birth. Overall the rate of pre-term deliveries in one study was 26.7 percent, and of these, 17.2 percent were single babies. Single IVF babies were also found to be at significant risk of being of low birth-weight: 11.5 percent weighed less than five and a half pounds.[25] Perinatal mortality rates for IVF and GIFT babies are three times higher than that of the general population[26] mainly due to prematurity and the increased number of multiple births, but there is also reported to be a higher incidence of spina bifida, transposition of the great vessels, and some forms of urinary tract malformation.

· *Julia* ·

My second child was an IVF baby. It took me several years to become pregnant with my first child and it was clear that it might take time again. I tried acupuncture with our practice nurse for four months first which didn't work, and then tried drugs. I decided I would have just one try at IVF before I was 40 and then if it didn't work we would just have to accept it and at least I wouldn't have regrets later in life that I hadn't tried it. We did, after all, have one healthy child.

My GP funded it and said, interestingly, that he had noticed that people got better results with the cheaper drugs and managed to call and get the drug prescription changed for me. I actually looked and felt better on them than I had on Clomid—the side effects did not prove as awful as I had feared. I made it quite clear that I would have only one attempt and I remember the technician saying to the consultant, "She's not coming back, you know, you'd better do it well," and laughing.

Fortunately it worked and I now have a lovely little boy.

Ectopic pregnancy

Ectopic pregnancy is a life-threatening condition which is on the increase. It is thought that one of the primary reasons for the rising numbers is due to the increase in pelvic inflammatory disease caused by sexually transmitted diseases such as chlamydia (see page 24), but it is also attributed to IVF and GIFT treatments and to the numbers of women having babies after the age of 35.

A pregnancy is ectopic if the fertilized egg implants outside the uterus, most commonly in the fallopian tubes. Although the embryo can be sustained there for a few weeks, it will eventually grow too big and cause the tube to rupture, causing serious internal bleeding, pain, and shock.

Symptoms prior to rupture can include vaginal bleeding, pain on one side, and possibly faintness. These signs in early pregnancy should be reported promptly for medical attention, particularly if they follow IVF, tubal surgery, or GIFT. Tubal rupture needs urgent surgical treatment to ensure the safety of the mother. In severe cases both the embryo and the tube may have to be removed. If it is detected before the tube ruptures, the condition may be managed conservatively, when it may be possible to save the tube, although not, unfortunately, the embryo. The options depend on the size of the embryo, how early it is detected, and whether there is any bleeding. It can be operated on laparoscopically or transvaginally, and can either involve opening the tube and restitching it, or injecting something into the embryo to kill it. As it is not uncommon for the embryo to die naturally and either be lost through the uterus and vagina, or reabsorbed, it may be possible to allow it to resolve naturally, provided close monitoring by means of blood, urine, and ultrasound is done.

The normal rate of ectopic pregnancy is 2 percent. This rises to 5 percent with assisted conception and as high as 60 percent if you have tubal surgery or have already had an ectopic pregnancy.

It is essential to get medical help immediately if there is any chance that you may be pregnant and have severe abdominal pain, particularly if it is one-sided, either with or without bleeding from the vagina.

You may need to insist on this, as ectopic pregnancy is sometimes not considered and diagnosed when it should be.

· *Gamete Intrafallopian* · *Transfer (GIFT)*

GIFT is similar to IVF in that eggs are gathered from a woman and mixed together with her partner's sperm outside her body. It differs in that the eggs and sperm are placed into her fallopian tubes immediately so that there is no way of knowing if they have fertilized. Its advantage is that the egg will travel down to the fallopian tube, taking several days, and so have the opportunity of implanting in the uterus in the normal time scale of five to seven days, instead of after two to three days, which is when embryos are placed into the uterus following IVF. Some authorities believe that GIFT has a higher success rate than IVF because it mimics the natural course of events more closely. The pregnancy rate is said to be higher, but this is subject to debate. In addition GIFT does involve a laparoscopy under general anesthetic, which can take some time, as the eggs are not only collected, but mixed with sperm and replaced in the fallopian tube.[27]

Who should have GIFT

Those with cervical factor hostility, endometriosis, or unexplained infertility.

Who should not have it

Women whose tubes are blocked or missing.

Short-term side effects

GIFT involves a general anesthetic, with its attendant risks, whereas IVF can be done vaginally, under sedation.

Long-term side effects

As for IVF (see page 50).

· *Superovulation With Intrauterine* · *Insemination (IUI)*

With this form of treatment ovulation is stimulated in women with unexplained infertility and apparently normal ovulation. The chances of conceiving are increased, either because of an increase in the number of follicles reaching maturity or because the treatment corrects some subtle defect in the ovulatory process. The chances of conception are then maximized by taking prepared sperm and inserting it directly into the uterus, bypassing the cervix. In one study, the success rate was said to be 6.8 percent, as opposed to 2.8 percent in women who were given a placebo instead of clomiphene.[28]

Side effects

As for Clomid. No continuing benefit has been demonstrated in trying superovulation and IUI for longer than six months and prolonged attempts are not recommended.

· *Other techniques* ·

ZIFT—zygote intrafallopian transfer
TET—tubal embryo transfer
PROST—pro-nuclear-stage transfer
POST—peritoneal oocycle sperm transfer

The above are refinements of the IVF technique, involving the removal of eggs, their fertilization outside the body and replacement at varying stages of development, but the fertilized eggs are returned to the fallopian tube rather than the uterus. These procedures are likely to require a general anesthetic and laparoscopy on two occasions in quick succession. At least one of the woman's fallopian tubes must be intact.

Side effects

As for IVF, but with the additional risk and side effects of general anesthesia.

4

COPING STRATEGIES

Infertility is undoubtedly a physical and emotional life crisis. As we saw in Chapter 2, it can create feelings of failure, worthlessness, abnormality and alienation, which can lead to anxiety, fear, shame and feelings of hopelessness and helplessness.[1]

Not surprisingly, many couples keep very quiet about something that makes them feel this way and may not share their experiences with, or gain support from, other couples in the same position. Therefore it may be useful to look at normal reactions to fertility problems and then to examine ways which other couples have found most helpful in dealing with their reactions.

Increasing the space between you and your problem

This may include withdrawing from painful situations, for example family occasions when children will be present, and avoiding pregnant women. The disadvantage of such strategies is that they can increase your sense of isolation, particularly as more of your friends have children, and it is not possible to avoid difficult situations altogether. They will always crop up, such as when a friend, a colleague, or a relation announces a pregnancy. Also, the more aware other people are that you find such situations hard to handle, the more likely they are to avoid the subject of children altogether, which in itself can lead to constraint between you, creating further loneliness.

You may find that drinking, smoking, taking tranquilizers or eating more makes you feel better, or you may take your feelings out on other people. Clearly these behaviors are not productive ways of coping. Eventually you will be able to adopt more positive strategies.

Making the problem of infertility less central and more peripheral includes getting involved with other activities and becoming very busy, taking up extra work and new interests, or spending more time on existing ones.

Regaining control

One of the things that people most dislike is the feeling of being out of control of their lives. You may find it useful to step aside from your situation for a while and make quite certain that you want to proceed with the next step. Be sure that it is your decision, rather than being led along from one thing to another. Becoming well informed about your problem will help you to feel that you have a better grip on the situation and that you are in charge. It can also help to get a clear treatment plan from your medical advisors, to decide what you want to happen, and ensure that it is done. The doctors are there to help you—that is their job and it is pointless agreeing to things that you feel are unnecessary or damaging. Equally, you may feel that they are doing each test in isolation when they should be getting the whole picture at once, or that something basic has been overlooked. Often a woman may undergo a whole battery of tests before her partner has even had a sperm sample assessed! It is perfectly reasonable to decide that you don't wish to pursue a particular course of action and the medical staff should support you in your decision.

Deciding to try a complementary medicine can increase your feeling of control. Appointments can be made at a time to suit you and the treatment has the added advantage of increasing your general health as well as being a means of improving your fertility. Taking control of your diet, weight, and level of exercise are other ways in which you can feel that you are doing something positive to help yourself.

Taking an active, problem-solving approach has helped many couples. For instance, some have lobbied for more recognition and funding for subfertility; others have worked to expand support networks, acting in the interests of both themselves and others in the same situation. Some couples find it helpful to make sure that the people treating them recognize the emotional aspects of subfertility and the impact that it has on them.

Being the best

It can help to improve your battered self-esteem if you aim to excel in at least one area. It might be personal appearance, fitness, work, diet—anything that increases your confidence and results in recognition that you are good at what you are doing. Some people have found that working hard to prevent sex from becoming mechanical is an achievement in which they can take pride.

Finding the hidden meaning

For some, convincing themselves that their problems exist for a reason or as part of a greater purpose is helpful. They may take comfort from the thought that their infertility must be God's will or that God has another plan for them. Others may be able to appreciate the areas of freedom that not having children gives them: not having to deal with diapers, not being tied to the house, being free to go out at will, eat out at leisure. Although you may resent these suggestions when made by other people, it can be helpful to realize that there is a positive side to childlessness.

Giving in to feelings

Some women describe crying in the shower and allowing feelings of intense sadness and bitterness to surface. One couple had a ritual which they followed when the woman's period started: she would ring her partner at work, then they would both leave work early; she would go home to bed while he picked up videotapes and chocolates before joining her in bed.

You may need outside help to enable you to discuss your feelings in depth with your partner. You or your partner may be protecting the other by not saying what you really feel. This can be just as true (or even more true) for seemingly united, loving couples as for those who find communication more difficult. It may be very hard to be completely honest if you feel your partner would be deeply hurt by what you say. Individual and joint counseling may provide the opportunity to air your feelings and this can be very liberating.

Sharing the burden

Many of the studies which have looked at the emotional problems relating to infertility have come to the same conclusion: the one thing that couples have found most helpful overall is a good social network—in other words, family and friends who provide support through an enduringly difficult time.

However, as we have seen, people also feel hurt when others make tactless remarks about their childlessness, offer unhelpful suggestions about ways of overcoming infertility, or suggest they are better off without children. Although, to a greater or lesser extent, these remarks are intended to help rather than to be unkind and may be born of ignorance, insensitivity, or a simple inability to empathize, they can be a serious deterrent to talking about the problem. Consequently, the whole matter can be driven underground, with the couple denying or refusing to admit to a problem when their families and friends could be supportive if given the opportunity.

It takes a lot of courage to disclose something you feel vulnerable about. It is hard to realize that other people will see your problem only as bad luck, not (as you may feel) as a reflection of your worth or your character, or as a punishment for something you did in the past. You may not want other people to follow your course of treatment or share your hopes and despairs with you, but the consensus seems to be that being open about fertility problems is helpful in the long run.

Support groups come into this category. Self-help groups can be very valuable because they work on the understanding that group members have some experience of what is under discussion. Therefore, you need not hold back for fear of upsetting anyone, or feel that the others do not really understand, never having been in your position, which may be true of friends and family. In itself this can be quite freeing, allowing you to laugh at or make fun of the horrors of your situation as well as to share the things that are especially painful. Some women have found it very encouraging to see others within the group becoming pregnant and moving on, offering them the hope that this can and does happen. Many women find that the experience of infertility hits them harder than their partners, and they may find it easier and more helpful to discuss their difficulties with other women rather than with their partners.

Whether you want people to believe that your childlessness is voluntary or involuntary will require explanation either way. It may be best to set the boundaries yourself, for example: "We are having some difficulty but I would rather not talk about it at the moment." You may decide who you will talk about it with, or be completely open. Openness is not easy, particularly if you feel the matter is a very private one, but it may be the least painful approach in the long run.

· *Shona* ·

I knew before we got married five years ago that I had problems with my tubes. When I was in college I got food poisoning very severely due to some undercooked chicken that was served in the residence hall. I was very ill but the doctor attributed it to my being three months pregnant, which I knew was an impossibility, and did not take the food poisoning seriously.

It has now been recognized that the damage to my tubes took place then, but at the time and for years afterwards I could not get anyone to take it seriously. It felt to me almost as if I had cancer; I had the same feeling of something eating its way through my body that my grandfather had while he was dying of cancer. Every time I moved and had a new doctor I would try to get it investigated, but no one would do anything as long as I was not actively trying for a baby. It took eighteen months to get a laparoscopy done and in the end I had it done privately, and found out just five weeks before my wedding that there was no viability in either of my tubes. The doctor who performed the laparoscopy was astounded that it had not been diagnosed before, but no one would do anything before it hit crisis point.

The following June we had our first attempt at IVF. It was very straightforward, apart from my developing very swollen ovaries, and three embryos were transplanted, but I didn't maintain the pregnancy.

In February 1994 we went for IVF again. On both occasions I produced sixteen eggs and this time we had six embryos. Three were replaced and three were cryopreserved. After I got back home I had bad stomach cramps as I was suffering from hyperstimulation. I was later taken back to the hospital, but they didn't find any free fluid; my body was just out of balance. I did not maintain the pregnancy this time either.

In the meantime I had been going to see a homeopath to relieve my sinus problems and asthma and stop the constant colds that I was getting. It worked very well, so that I have hardly ever had to use my inhaler since, and it was a wonderful therapy which made me feel a lot better. I also started seeing an acupuncturist in order to prepare me for the IVF treatment. I found it wonderfully calming and both the acupuncture and the homeopathy made me feel a million times better and much more robust.

In April 1996 I went back to hospital to have the embryos replaced. I was under drug control to make sure that the timing was absolutely accurate and it went very straightforwardly; I had no side effects but I did not maintain the pregnancy.

At the beginning of December, at around the time my period would have been due, I started to feel very unwell. I was very busy and working too hard. I did start to wonder if I might be pregnant but I live in a very small community and I didn't want to buy a pregnancy test because everyone would have known about it. I also thought that it might be a phantom pregnancy, so I kept putting off the test.

Then one day I collapsed at work. My doctor was very reluctant to visit me at all, but when he did said that I had a virus and gave me pain-killers. I was in agony, so much so that my husband thought that I was dying. We called the doctor again. By this time I was lying on the bathroom floor screaming in pain and vomiting. He gave me pethidine and said that either he or another doctor *would call the next day but that we were to cancel the appointment if I felt better before then. Fortunately the doctor who called the next day took me to the hospital immediately. By this time I could no longer speak and I was close to the edge. They did various tests and thought that it might be kidney failure at first but then they came to me and said, "you are very pregnant." I knew then that I was in desperate trouble and that I had been bleeding internally for over a week. They got me into the operating room in a panic with the anesthetist shouting at me to keep my oxygen mask on. They found litres of blood in my abdominal cavity; my right tube had contained an eight- to nine-week old baby and had ruptured. They had to remove the baby and the tube. It was an awful end.*

After this I started to see a reflexologist, who was someone I already knew and trusted. The treatment that she gave me was wonderful and gave me a real sense of well-being and made me feel so much better. However, she told me that she could feel something in my left tube (the right one had been removed). I really thought that she was a quack at this point and that she didn't know her job, but she turned out to be absolutely right. There was some debris left over from the ectopic pregnancy in the tube which made it very distended, swollen and sore. I had to go back to hospital and have an emergency laparotomy and tubal surgery in order to clear it.

The whole experience has changed me—it has really toughened me up. I'm much more aware of my needs and those of other people now, and I will no longer let them ride roughshod over me. It has made me a more rounded, better person and we have the satisfaction of knowing that we have the resilience to withstand these things. It has been awful, but lots of people have tragedies in their lives and don't let them stand in their way. I don't want to be an 80- or 90-year-old with lots of regrets, and I feel that reflexology has been very useful in reducing stress levels so that we can look forward.

Interestingly, although I would not have credited that I would have felt that way, having the ectopic pregnancy has made me feel much more of a woman. You can feel that you have very little self-worth and as if you are not quite whole, a bit sub-human if you need intervention. People treat you as if you are a bit strange if you need IVF, but now that we've managed it ourselves without any intervention they treat us differently. I feel a huge change in myself because I know I've had a natural pregnancy.

· *Marianne* ·

We tried for our first child for six and a half years until I finally made the decision to stop trying. By that time we had been through an awful lot and I decided that it was taking over our lives. It put a lot of pressure on us; my husband felt it quite strongly and it had affected our sex life so that we reached a point where he would say, "Is it tonight?" and I'd say "Yes" and he would say, "Oh no!" because after a busy day and in a demanding job it was the last thing he felt like. When I made the decision to stop trying it took the pressure off, neither of us had to perform at a set time. We were fed up with the disappointment every month, but I had read about the disadvantages of medical procedures and didn't want to get involved with them. I felt that enough was enough and that we had been married a long time.

When I first became aware of the problem I did a temperature chart for six months and then took it to one of the obstetric guys at work to see if he could figure out when I was ovulating, if anywhere, because it wasn't easy to read. He was so rude to me, wouldn't help and said, "These things are a waste of time." So we abandoned that and I was referred to a hospital. They tested my husband, who was fine; we did a post-coital test, which was fine and a laparoscopy and dye, which in theory was absolutely fine too. They just said "Everything is fine—go away and practice." I suppose I should have been more assertive, and asked what happens next, but they assured us that everything was all right. It was to be another two years before we conceived.

I did try Clomid and tamoxifen for four months each. I felt awful on Clomid and lost lots of weight although I was eating the same amount of food, and everyone commented how awful I looked. I had a dreadful pallor and my hair went very limp and I just did not feel a hundred percent. They persisted longer with the drugs because they knew that I wouldn't try anything else.

I left my job as a nurse and took a year off to do a course at a university. That removed the stress of the job, but I still did not become pregnant. At the end I decided to concentrate on my career and got a new and more senior position. Within seven to eight months I was pregnant.

I became pregnant at the New Year, staying away in a hotel. I did have an inkling that it might have been a good time, although my husband did not, but I never for a moment dreamed that it would work. We could not believe it when it turned out that I really was pregnant. We had been through so many disappointments of being late and having raised hopes before, so that it was a good seven weeks before I actually did a test. The delight when it proved positive was overwhelming! It fitted in beautifully with the job, too, which I wasn't enjoying. I went back briefly when my daughter was born and was happy to stop.

I think perhaps there was a contributing factor. My younger sister died very suddenly after we had been married for two years, and a lot of people put pressure on us to have a family as a consequence. I knew that wasn't right for my parents, my mother in particular wasn't ready, it took her quite a few years to get over it and I think perhaps I wasn't ready psychologically.

5

IMPROVING YOUR CHANCES OF NATURAL CONCEPTION

· *Diet* ·

Food and drink really do matter if you are trying to conceive, not only for conception but to maintain a healthy pregnancy. It can be hard to take the necessary steps to improve your diet if you are not convinced of the value of doing it or if the things that you enjoy are on the "forbidden" list. You may feel that they console you for not becoming pregnant and that it is bad enough restricting your diet for the sake of the baby if you do conceive, but awful to have to go without some of life's pleasures and not be pregnant either. You will almost certainly know one or more couples who are overweight, smoke, and eat only manufactured foods, and yet are superfertile, which will not help.

It is tempting to rationalize your intake as being the best you can manage in the circumstances, but diet is the first area to consider and the one over which you do have control. If you are not already living your life along the healthy guidelines currently advised, you may want to sit down and consider where it could be improved. It may be that old patterns of eating and drinking have caused underlying deficiencies which you may need supplements to overcome. The effect of nutrition on fertility is still not fully understood and it is becoming clearer that food and its additives, together with the pesticides and herbicides used in modern agricultural practices, are playing a considerable part in infertility, and particularly in falling sperm counts.

Perhaps the best way to review your joint diets is to write a meticulous food diary for a week, recording everything you eat and drink—including the things you might want to gloss over. Also work out your total fluid intake daily. There is strong evidence, for example, that fertility can be substantially reduced by caffeine; your intake may be easily raised if you work in an office where percolated coffee is always available. Once you have a typical week's intake to study you will be able to see where you might make changes in the food you buy, how you decide what to eat and drink, and how you prepare food.

You may find that this means more of your time is taken up with food preparation, particularly if the only way to eat and drink well during the day is to take your own supplies with you to work. Fresh food is better for you than manufactured food—even though it is far easier just to put something into the microwave. Although manufactured foods may provide balanced meals, they contain preservatives and other chemicals designed to improve the keeping quality of the product. These substances have been passed as being of food quality and standard and are not known to cause overt poisoning, but it is quite possible that the cumulative effect of additives and preservatives may affect your fertility. People react individually to food and the things manufacturers put into them.

It may be that a food you are particularly fond of, and which you eat frequently, can be causing problems. It need not be manufactured: often apparently wholesome food, such as dairy products or citrus fruit, causes a reaction in someone who craves them. The craving can be part of the symptoms, other aspects of the reaction being hard to link to the food.

It can be a challenge to revise your diet in this way, trying to decide where, if anywhere, you need to make changes. Clearly, it still has to be tailored to your likes and dislikes, but it is valuable to introduce as much variety as possible, making sure that food is freshly prepared whenever you can. It may be a good idea to cook meals at weekends and store them in the freezer. Cook in large quantities, separating the food into batches, including some single person portions for the times when you are not eating together. It is easy to make do with something quick and not especially nutritious if you are alone. If you take frozen food out of the freezer the night before and leave it in the fridge, it can be heated quickly the following evening.

· *Nadia* ·

I had always had normal periods and conceived my first child straightaway. After he was six months old I stopped breast-feeding him and my periods returned. They were unlike anything that I had ever experienced before, much longer and very painful with brown bleeding. I couldn't understand what was happening and no one gave me an explanation or diagnosed it. It was when my son was about three and we wanted another child and I found that I could not conceive that I started to get really concerned. I hadn't thought that I could have a fertility problem as I had not found it difficult before, but as time went by I began to get desperate.

I happened to discuss it with a friend of mine whose daughter-in-law just had a radical hysterectomy for her endometriosis and she said, "That's what you've got." I managed to get an appointment with a gynecologist and he found that I did have endometriosis very badly and that my tubes were starting to become blocked. I can only surmise that I had acquired it as a result of surgical transplantation when my son was born as an emergency cesarean. I was very upset as I could see my hopes of having another child disappearing.

I started taking a multivitamin, although nothing else, and joined the Endometriosis Association (see Useful Addresses). I refused to take any drugs for the endometriosis and eventually decided to see a alternative health consultant. He diagnosed me as having systemic candida and put me on a diet. He told me what I should not eat but not why I shouldn't eat it and didn't provide any explanations, leaving it up to his nurse to back up his consultation. He was not at all approachable and was very expensive and distant. I tried the diet and intravenous infusions and I felt that it may have helped a little, but then I started to get flooding with my periods so I was ultimately worse off.

I knew from the Endometriosis Association that some women with endometriosis had been helped by being on a macrobiotic diet, so I consulted someone about trying it. He put me on a dreadful radical diet. I really wanted it to work, so I followed it to the letter. It did work, in that the pain stopped, but so did my periods. I lost an awful lot of weight and found the diet very hard going. I became so obsessed about the food that I couldn't eat and I was still having to cook normally for my family.

After four months I just snapped. I smelled something nice and went berserk and ate everything that I could find. I went bulimic and was in complete despair because I felt that the diet had been my last chance of having a baby. Eventually I phoned a nutritional consultant associated with the Endometriosis Association in tears one day. She was wonderful and so helpful—she said I could phone her at any time and she spent hours with me talking me through my problems and sorted me out nutritionally. She took me off the macrobiotic diet and put me on something that was not too radical although taking out the bad things. I continued to take my vitamins and minerals (and had done so while on the macrobiotic diet, although they had told me I shouldn't) and I also started to take zinc and vitamin C and something that she prescribed to help me digest my food. We stopped eating anything that was manufactured and found that organic food tasted so much better and fresher. I started to feel much better and had a lot more energy. I had a light period and after that I became pregnant. I took the vitamins all through the pregnancy and had no problems. My son was born by elective cesarean at 38 weeks and weighed around 7$\frac{1}{2}$ pounds. They had a look at the time of the operation and found that there was only a small amount of the endometriosis left.

By this time the diet had become a way of life. I now hardly ever drink coffee or eat chocolate, but when I do it makes me feel dreadfully tired, so I usually drink herbal tea. I felt so much better that I was not really surprised to find that I had become pregnant again, this time with our daughter. She is two now. I breast-fed her for a year and my periods returned a year ago and are entirely back to normal. She was born by elective cesarean as well and this time they said all the endometriosis had gone.

Two of my friends who had great problems conceiving finally managed to conceive (one at 43 with donor eggs) once they were convinced that diet really does matter. I was on the point of trying IVF when I finally got good advice. The gynecologist that I saw said that diet didn't make any difference. I am so grateful to the

*nutritionist for helping me to prove him wrong. She was so good at
telling me why things would make a difference. We are all ignorant
to start with and it is only with knowledge that you can help yourself.*

· *Guidelines for healthy eating* ·

1. Reduce your intake of sugar and refined carbohydrates as far
   as possible. These include sugar, candies, biscuits, cakes,
   chocolates, puddings, jam, honey, glucose, ice cream, soft
   drinks, and other sweet foods. Many also contain refined
   flour which is low in vitamins and minerals, and may have a
   surprisingly high salt content. It is best to eat whole grain
   bread whenever possible.
2. Reduce your intake of animal and vegetable fats. Most people
   have a diet that is high in fat, but some foods, such as dairy
   products, may be high in fat and yet provide other benefits,
   whereas others, particularly manufactured foods, have high
   levels of animal fats but relatively low nutritional values, for
   example, sausages, pies, canned meats, cakes, and cookies.
3. Eat plenty of fruits and vegetables—five generous portions a
   day are considered desirable. Vegetables should be cooked
   only lightly and organic produce is definitely preferable. A
   steamer makes cooking vegetables easier and helps to preserve the vitamins within them instead of losing them to the
   water they are boiled in.

   You might be able to reduce the amount of pesticides you
   take in by washing or peeling fruit and vegetables, but many
   pesticides are systemic, which means that the whole plant is
   treated and the chemicals are inside the fruit or vegetable.
   Nutritional experts suggest that when you are unable to
   obtain organic produce, fruit and vegetables are probably
   best bought from large supermarket chains where methods
   of farming the produce they buy are kept under closer super-
   vision than may be the case elsewhere. A study by Danish
   scientists showed that sperm samples taken from members of
   the Danish Association of Organic Farmers, 25 percent of

whose diet consisted of pesticide-free produce, contained 43 percent more sperm that that taken from men of similar age who worked for an airline.

4. It is important to eat a reasonable amount of fiber, including legumes, fruits, vegetables, cereals and wholegrain bread. Fiber has the benefit of providing more bulk in the gut, speeding the passage of waste material through it, and thus reducing the chance of developing cancer of the large bowel. Fruits and vegetables also include beta-carotene, which helps fight free radicals (see page 78).

   However, be aware of how and when you include fiber in your diet. Some types of fiber, especially bran or that produced by the fiber content of wheat, contain phytic acid, which can bind to iron and zinc in the diet, forming insoluble compounds which are excreted, thus losing the benefit of the food eaten and increasing the chances of becoming iron or zinc deficient. This is of particular significance because deficiencies of both have been linked with infertility. Zinc deficiency especially is associated with hypogonadism (underactivity of the testes) and is more common in vegetarians, who may be eating large quantities of foods containing phytates and failing to absorb the zinc in their diets. They may, in any case, not be consuming much zinc as it is more readily found in meat and shellfish than plant sources.

5. Keep alcohol consumption low—this applies to both men and women. Alcohol can affect sperm by reducing its production, while acetaldehyde, one of the breakdown products of alcohol metabolism, is toxic to sperm. Alcohol also interferes with testosterone secretion and speeds up its breakdown within the body, hastening its conversion to estrogen. High levels of estrogen in men significantly lower sperm counts and are also responsible for the feminization of their appearance (as with the beer belly and over-developed breasts noticeable in some male drinkers). Drinking can also be responsible for excess weight gain, which can, if severe, result in fat which surrounds the testes, raising the temperature above that in which they can function (see page 99).

Alcohol is advised against when trying to conceive, less because it may prevent conception (although some women with long-standing fertility problems have become pregnant when they gave up even a low consumption of alcohol completely), but also because it may affect the embryo in the very early days even before a positive pregnancy test. Interesting and reasoned debate on the risks of alcohol in pregnancy is contained in Judy Priest's book *Drugs in Conception, Pregnancy and Childbirth* (see Further Reading). She points out that alcohol prohibition in pregnancy is a relatively new phenomenon and that it is unlikely that low levels of less than 10 units a week will do any harm provided the drinking is spread over several days and not drunk all the time. One unit is:

One shot of spirits
One glass of wine
One bottle of beer

However, you may feel happier if you avoid alcohol altogether during the second half of your cycle. Some would say that any drinking around the time of conception is harmful but there is no evidence for this. There is evidence though, that heavy drinking in pregnancy can cause fetal alcohol syndrome in the baby, which may be responsible for facial deformities and mental retardation. Alcohol may also increase the chance of miscarrying if taken in large quantities.

6. If you are either over or under weight (see pages 84–87), you may need to take steps to correct it. Excess weight in men and both low weight and obesity in women can cause fertility problems.

7. Try to drink 8 glasses of water every day. It is easy to become dehydrated in a work environment.

Some of the dietary recommendations given above are discussed elsewhere in the book, while others, such as smoking (also mentioned on page 91), are concerned with lifestyle rather than diet, yet may have a direct bearing on fertility.

Caffeine

Perhaps surprisingly, caffeine has been shown to have a dramatic effect on fertility in women. Several studies have shown that caffeine intake can substantially lengthen the time it takes to become pregnant. One trial which involved 1,430 women who were trying to become pregnant showed that the consumption of more than 300 mg of caffeine daily almost tripled the likelihood of not becoming pregnant within twelve months and reduced the monthly chance by 26 percent compared with women who did not consume caffeine.[1] They estimated caffeine intake by allotting the following values to these drinks :

> One cup of caffeinated coffee: 100 mg
> One cup of tea: 50 mg
> One can of soft drink (e.g. Coke): 40 mg

Only two cups of coffee and four cups of tea daily will put you over the 300 mg limit and seriously affect your chances of conceiving. A previous study,[2] which also selected women who were planning to become pregnant, reported a 50 percent decrease in the probability rate of pregnancy among women who tried for three months or more to become pregnant when they were consuming as little as one cup of coffee a day.

This very powerful contraceptive effect is explained by some of the actions that caffeine has. It is known to cause DNA damage,[3] and to be a neuroendocrine and cardiovascular stimulant. The rate at which caffeine is excreted is dependent on the menstrual cycle. It is cleared from the body more slowly during the luteal phase (the second half), so that there is a greater amount within the body at the time when the embryo would be implanting and starting to develop.[4] Moreover, it has been shown that caffeine can lead to miscarriage in both humans and animals, so that it could be responsible for early losses, thus extending the apparent time before pregnancy occurs. According to several trials, it can also lead to lowered birth-weight. Clearly, it is a good idea to reduce caffeine levels to below that of 300 mg.

· *Vitamins and minerals* ·

There is always some debate as to whether vitamin and mineral supplements are necessary and desirable for women planning pregnancy. Some experts feel that most people eat a good diet which is unlikely to leave them short of any vitamins. Others feel that poor health, stress, exhaustion, or having taken the pill can leave women depleted of vitamins and minerals so that they should at least take a multivitamin.

As already discussed, some couples and women in particular, do not eat well—either too much or too little or the wrong sort of food. If you are having problems conceiving, it is possible that one (or both) of you is either not consuming or not retaining the right balance of proteins, carbohydrates or fats; alternatively you may be getting too little or too much of some vitamins, minerals, or trace elements. Your diet may not be at fault at all; it is possible that some inborn error of metabolism, or something about the environment in which you live or the conditions under which you work can cause these problems. For example, a man with a low sperm count who works in a boiler room might be low in zinc, because excessive sweating increases loss of zinc. It could also be that the exposure to heat raises the temperature in his testes, or it could be due to a combination of both these and other factors.

It is not necessarily easy to eat well or to find and afford organic food, although you can grow your own. It is possible that you could be eating a diet rich in fruit and vegetables, but taking in unacceptable levels of pesticides, or that the produce, although beautiful in appearance, has little flavor, suggesting that it has been artificially ripened (that is particularly likely with imported fruit and vegetables), so that it has not been allowed to ripen in the sun and develop its full quota of vitamins.

For all of these reasons it may be necessary to take supplements. There is plenty of research to show that vitamins and minerals are implicated as being necessary for reproduction and that lack of them can cause infertility in some cases. More evidence is being published all the time, although it may not be accepted by some doctors working in the field of human reproduction. Some women report their doctors as being skeptical or scathing about the effect diet or supplements can have on conception.

The best advice on supplements that can improve sperm counts in men and improve reproductive health in women can be found in Dr. Stephen Davies and Dr. Alan Stewart's excellent book, *Nutritional Medicine* (see Further Reading). This book contains over 500 pages of detailed information on the effects that nutrition has on the biochemistry of our bodies and how we can repair them through diet and mineral supplements rather than drugs.

The following suggestions for supplements for men and women are those recommended by Davies and Stewart, backed up by further research carried out since their book was published.

Supplements for men

Studies have shown that taking nutritional supplements can improve sperm counts. It is certainly important not to take too much, as selenium for example, can impair fertility both when you take too much as well as too little. Nutrients that are essential for normal sperm formulation include:

Essential fatty acids

Essential fatty acids (EFAs) are known to be essential for gonadal functioning in experimental animals and it seems likely that this is true of humans too. The prostaglandins in semen are derived from essential fatty acids, and some men with unexplained infertility have low levels of seminal prostaglandins. Essential fatty acids supplements also help schizophrenics, people who bruise easily, and those with eczema, dry skin and dandruff, brittle nails, frequent infections, inflammatory conditions, such as rheumatoid and other forms of arthritis, some kidney diseases, certain blood clotting problems, angina, multiple sclerosis, premenstrual syndrome (PMS), benign breast disease, diabetes, obesity, dry eyes, and Raynaud's phenomenon.

You might be deficient in EFAs if your hair is falling out, if you have dandruff, eczema or poor wound healing, are unusually sweaty, very thirsty, or have fertility problems (especially men), kidney problems, dry eyes and lack of saliva, depigmentation of skin (lighter patches) or loss of muscle tone, if you bruise easily, have mental disturbances, poor vision, heart abnormalities, diarrhea, bronchial disorders or pimples like goose-flesh on upper arms, thighs, and buttocks.

Although it might not be apparent, other signs of EFA deficiency include impaired cholesterol transport, pancreas gland withering, and fatty degeneration of the liver. In these cases, you should reduce your intake of animal fats and consume more polyunsaturated oil and plenty of vegetables, salads, nuts, and seeds. Avoid alcohol, smoking, and refined carbohydrates.

The recommended dose for adults is

1–4 g evening primrose oil
4–8 capsules fish oil

These should not be taken if you have epilepsy or a bleeding disorder.

Zinc

Zinc is essential for reproduction in both men and women. Zinc deficiency has been found to be responsible for low sperm counts in some men (and also impotence). In studies where such men took zinc, they found their levels raised to normal after three months and their testosterone levels rose, too. Anecdotally, zinc supplementation has helped many overcome infertility.

You may be deficient in zinc if you have infertility, low sperm count, hair loss, various skin conditions, diarrhea, immune deficiencies, sleep and behavioral disturbances, night blindness, impaired taste or smell, find wounds heal slowly or have white spots on your fingernails (often thought, mistakenly, to be due to calcium deficiency).

Certain groups of people are more likely to be zinc deficient; these include those who are anorexic, are dieting, (especially those on bizarre diets), on exclusion diets for allergies, vegetarians and particularly vegans, those who eat soy substitutes for meat, alcoholics, and the elderly.

It is thought that as food has become more refined, many more people are at risk of zinc deficiency. In addition, certain other foods can interfere with its absorption—zinc taken at the same time as iron supplements may mean that the zinc is not absorbed by the body. There are foods that should not be taken within an hour of taking the supplement. They include soy protein, soy milk foods, coffee, cow's milk, chocolate, hamburgers, celery, lemon, brown bread, wholewheat bread, high-fiber diet foods, and bran.

As already mentioned high-fiber foods, especially wheat, can bind with available zinc to form insoluble compounds which are excreted.

Zinc is found in: oysters, ginger root, muscle meats (lamb chops and steak), pecans, split peas, Brazil nuts, beef liver, non-fat dry milk, egg yolk, wholewheat, rye, oats, peanuts, lima beans, soy lecithin, almonds, walnuts, chicken, buckwheat, hazelnuts, clams, green peas, shrimps, turnips, parsley, potatoes, garlic, wholewheat bread, carrots, beans, raw milk, pork chops, and corn.

Supplement: 50 mg elemental zinc a day.

Chromium

Chromium is essential for sperm formation. Although only very small amounts are present in the body, it is thought to be required for controling blood sugar level, and it is essential for the action of insulin and maintenance of normal blood sugar. Lower-than-average levels of chromium can lead to diabetes and arteriosclerosis. One of the other effects is to depress sperm formation.

Chromium is found in: brewer's yeast, black pepper, calf's liver, wheat germ, wholewheat bread, and cheese.

Supplement: 200 mg a day.

Selenium

There is no doubt that selenium is necessary for normal sperm formation and, while it is possible to have too much of it, recent research shows that intake of selenium in Britain and Europe is decreasing.

Selenium is important for sperm formation because sperm capsule selenoprotein is found in the mid-piece region of the sperm tail. Selenium deficiency gives rise to sperm with impaired fertility; it is also needed for normal testosterone metabolism and testicular morphology. Several other selenoproteins are found in the testes. In a double-blind trial, sperm fertility improved from 17.5 percent to 35.1 percent in subfertile men supplemented with selenium.[5]

Another study showed that British intakes of selenium have fallen from 60 mcg a day 22 years ago to 34 mcg a day currently. This is substantially lower than current recommended intakes (75 mcg for men and 60 mcg for women) and the reason is thought to be due to EU levies; the British no longer import North American high-protein wheat which is rich in selenium.

This problem is less critical in the United States, but there is still cause for concern because the bioavailability of selenium in plant material has declined due to acid rain and excessive artificial fertilization of soil.[6]

Selenium is found in: Brazil nuts (the richest natural source), grains, fish, and most whole foods.

Supplement: 100 to 200 mcg (this should always be taken together with vitamin E).

Warning: Selenium levels of 800 mcg and above are toxic. Be especially careful if you think you may already be taking too much selenium, which is possible if you work in or live close to smelting works, work in the production of glass and ceramics, rubber, steel and brass, paint and paint pigments, or plastics, or in a photo-electrical chemical industry.

Vitamin E

Vitamin E is essential for reproduction. It has been recognized for thousands of years that animals that are deficient in vitamin E are unable to have successful pregnancies.

Vitamin E protects against the damaging effects that oxygen and other oxidizing substances can have on living tissues. These free radicals, as they are known, can seriously damage the structure of cell membranes and the contents of living cells. Accelerated damage can lead to cell death.

Superoxide free radicals are found in semen, produced by white blood cells and from the manufacture of sperm.[7] It is possible to have semen tested to detect the level of free radicals as high levels can be responsible for subfertility, although this is not done routinely.

Antioxidants will protect against oxydizing free-radical attacks, so taking vitamin E (200 mg three times a day), together with vitamin C (1 g four times a day), is recommended, particularly for those who have identified this problem. Vitamin E should always be taken with selenium.

Vitamin E also helps maintain the flexibility of sperm cell walls, which is needed for motility and helps prevent the sperm from clumping together.

Vitamin E is found in: vegetable oils, nuts, seeds, soy products, lettuce, eggs, wheat germ, and dairy products.

Vitamin C

Low levels of vitamin C, which is also an antioxidant, can cause problems with fertility. Men who have been on diets containing less than 250 mg daily have been shown to have sperm which were clumped together; their sperm also had damaged DNA (genetic defects). Vitamin C has an antioxidant effect on its own but it also helps to maintain vitamin E in a nonoxidized form and therefore helps to prevent clumping.

The dose recommended above (1 g four times a day) is a high one, and should be taken with caution if you or your family have a history of kidney stones. Long-term administration can also reduce the availability of trace elements such as copper and zinc. However, vitamin C does have the advantage of reducing lead and cadmium levels in the body and can be useful in eliminating heavy metals from the body.

You can either ask for free-radical levels in sperm to be checked or take it as suggested and see whether it helps. In trials, the beneficial effect of vitamin C supplementation—or the damaging effects of reducing it—began to be seen within a week, but full spermatogenesis takes around 70 days.

Vitamin C is found in: Fruits, green vegetables, liver, cabbage, and potatoes.

Vitamin B

The B vitamins are important in sex-hormone metabolism and libido. They have been shown to be necessary for male fertility in animals.

Thiamin (vitamin B_1) is found in: whole grains, pork, beef, peas, beans, lentils, and brown rice.

Riboflavin (vitamin B_2) is found in: milk and other dairy products, cereals, meats, and some green leafy vegetables.

Niacin or nicotinic acid (vitamin B_3) is found in: meat, beef, milk, fish, and whole grains.

Pantothenic acid (vitamin B_5) is found in: eggs, whole-grain cereals, and meat.

Pyridoxine (vitamin B_6) is found in: meats, fish, egg yolk, whole grain cereals, bananas, avocados, nuts, seeds, and some green leafy vegetables.

Vitamin B_{12} is found in: liver and other organ meats, meat, fish, dairy products, eggs, and brewer's yeast.

Vitamin A

Vitamin A is also involved in maintaining the stability of cell membranes. It is found in animal produce and beta-carotene, a vitamin A-type compound. It is found in the yellow pigments of vegetables—any green, yellow, or orange-colored fruit or vegetable.

Beta-carotene is the best-absorbed receptor of the damaging free-radicals. If it is not needed, it remains as beta-carotene; if needed, it is converted into vitamin A.

Vitamin A is found in: animal and fish livers, kidneys, eggs, milk, and butter.

Food sources of beta-carotene: carrots, spinach, cabbage, and orange and yellow fruits.

Amino acids

Stewart and Davies also recommend taking supplements of free-form amino acids—500 mg of the major amino acids twice daily.

Amino acids are needed in the formation of the building blocks of protein which are essential for growth and in the replacement of body parts. They are also needed for the production of chemicals and hormones.

Amino acids are contained in first-class proteins—meat, fish, eggs, and dairy products. Vegetarian proteins are second-class proteins which contain amino acids but they are not complete, so that they need to be mixed to provide all the essential amino acids.

Arginine is an amino acid which is found in unusually high quantities in the head of the sperm. **Lysine**, another amino acid is also thought to be of value in maintaining male fertility. The recommended dose for each is 500 mg a day.

Supplements for women

Stewart and Davies recommend the following preconceptional vitamin and mineral supplements:

vitamin E	100–200 IUs
vitamin A	2500–5000 IUs
vitamin C	100–500 mg
vitamins B_1, B_2, B_3, B_6	2–20 mg
vitamin B_{12}	200–300 mcg
choline	10–20 mg
inositol	10–20 mg
folic acid	400–800 mcg
zinc	10–20 mg
manganese	5–10 mg
calcium	400–800 mg
copper	0.5–1 mg
iron	10–20 mg
selenium	25–50 mg

Most of these can be obtained in one multivitamin and mineral tablet, although it is important to check the exact figures.

No woman planning pregnancy should take more than 5,000 IUs of vitamin A as a supplement, as there is a risk that excessive doses of this vitamin could cause fetal malformations.

Supplements for post-pill recovery

Stewart and Davies believe that taking the pill causes nutritional deficiencies which may be responsible for failure to menstruate and ovulate when a woman stops taking the pill. They consider that it increases circulating levels of vitamin A, but interferes with the metabolism of vitamins B_1, B_2, B_6, B_{12}, and folic acid. Low folate levels are clearly associated with a rise in the number of neural tube defects in babies, such as spina bifida and anencephaly.

Vitamin C requirements are increased by taking the pill and should be supplemented by 500 mg while taking it. (Taking more can convert a low-dose pill into a high-dose one.) Vitamin D remains unchanged, but vitamin E levels drop by about 20 percent while taking the pill. It is recommended to take vitamins A and B_6 while on the pill—see the list below.

Copper levels increase while on the pill and in pregnancy, zinc levels are lowered, but iron levels remain the same (because there is less bleeding). In the authors" experience the pill also causes a magnesium deficiency.

For post-pill recovery a healthy diet is essential, together with the following recommended supplements:

vitamin B_1	10–50 mg
vitamin B_2	10–50 mg
vitamin B_3	10–50 mg
vitamin B_5	50–100 mg
vitamin B_6	50–100 mg
vitamin B_{12}	200–400 mcg
folic acid	400 mcg–2mg

inositol	50–75 mg
choline	50–75 mg
vitamin A	not necessary
vitamin C	250–2000 mg (or more)
vitamin E	50–200 IUs
magnesium	100–200 mg (or more)
zinc	5–15 mg (or more)
manganese	3–5 mg
copper	not necessary
iron	depends on status

Premenstrual syndrome, heavy periods, and dysmenorrhea (difficult and painful periods) may also be helped by taking supplements. If your periods are heavy, you may need to take them for two to three months before an improvement is seen.

Premenstrual syndrome

Follow the dietary suggestions on page 68, making sure to restrict sugars, salts, red meat and alcohol, stop smoking, reduce your intake of fats, especially animal fats and saturated fats. If you crave sweets and chocolates, eat high-quality protein snacks.

Take a multivitamin with 100 mg B_6 daily plus B vitamins and vitamin C, or vitamin B_6, 100–200 mg alone. Many women find B_6 helpful but a more balanced supplement is preferable; evening primrose oil, 2-4 g a day, either two weeks before the period or throughout the cycle; vitamin E 300, 500 IUs a day, and magnesium, 200-300 mg elemental magnesium a day.

Painful periods

Take calcium, magnesium, vitamin E, zinc and EFAs (see page 73). The improvement may take place over several months.

Heavy periods

Take iron, zinc, vitamin B_6, vitamin A, and bioflavanoids.

Iron

Iron deficiencies may play a significant part in female infertility, although this is not commonly recognized. Iron deficiency can occur even in the absence of anemia, and women, especially those who have heavy periods or are strict vegetarians are particularly at risk. Iron deficiency is said to be very common and underdiagnosed. Symptoms can include listlessness, tiredness, rapid heartbeat in response to moderate exercise, sore tongue, cracks at the corners of the mouth, and concave nails. It may also be responsible for poor hair growth.

A group of 113 women between the ages of 18 and 54 who were being treated at a London trichology clinic for hair loss, were almost all found to have low levels of ferritin (molecules which carry iron in the blood). They were given a daily dose of 35 mg iron and 200 mg of vitamin C to counteract their iron deficiency and improve their hair growth. Within 28 weeks, seven who had previously had fertility problems became pregnant, including a 42-year-old who had had nine years of failed fertility treatment.[8] Obviously, this is of significance only to women with low ferritin levels; these can be checked by a blood test done by your GP.

If your ferritin levels are low, and you want to take iron supplements, it is important that you are careful as to how you take them, as certain foods and minerals can prevent them from being absorbed. Iron absorption is impaired by whole grains, soy, and legumes. It is also decreased if tea or coffee is taken at the same time as iron, either from dietary sources or iron supplements. Tea or coffee can be drunk an hour before a meal, but if it is taken with a meal or one and a half to two hours later, it can decrease the amount of iron absorbed by as much as 64 percent. Tea is more damaging than coffee.

If you are taking zinc supplements, they should be separated from the iron supplements by several hours as zinc interferes with iron absorption, too. As meals can also prevent zinc absorption, the zinc should be taken an hour or more before or after meals.

Vitamin C helps to promote iron absorption.

· *Carol* ·

We tried for years to have a baby—we started trying in 1990. I didn't become pregnant and after a laparoscopy I was told that I had mild endometriosis and a retroverted womb, but that this shouldn't prevent my becoming pregnant, so the diagnosis was really unexplained infertility. I went to my GP, who prescribed Clomid for six months, but nothing happened. I don't know whether or not I was ovulating, but I didn't become pregnant. We then had superovulation, which was not successful.

We were put on a waiting list for IUI and while we were waiting for the appointment, we tried IVF privately. The first time that they did it, they abandoned the cycle because I didn't produce any suitable eggs. The second time I was put on the highest possible dosage of drugs to stimulate egg production, but I only produced four and it didn't work. We then had the IUI we were waiting for and had three attempts.

After that we happened to attend a talk at the hospital we were going to. The speaker talked about various vitamins and minerals that might help. We felt that taking supplements couldn't do any harm so dashed out and bought some zinc and selenium, which were the ones that she had particularly mentioned.

After six months I was pregnant. Unfortunately, I miscarried at ten weeks but, although it was very distressing, I also felt that it was hopeful because I had at least gotten pregnant. After the miscarriage I started taking the tablets again. This time I also visited an alternative therapist, who recommended that we also take B vitamins, folic acid, vitamin E, calcium and magnesium, oil of evening primrose, and bioflavanoids.

I became pregnant again after six months. Although I was concerned about taking the vitamins while I was pregnant, I continued to take them. I did have quite a bit of bleeding for which I took progesterone. There are so many ifs and buts that you can never be sure exactly what worked, but I think that it was the zinc that really helped. I always used to get cold sores, but I haven't had them anything like as badly or as often since I've been taking zinc. I took 14 mgs a day throughout pregnancy—I did get morning sickness, but not badly, and I felt it was a good sign. The only other thing I did to help become pregnant was douche with approximately half a teaspoon of bicarbonate of soda, although there had been no evidence of cervical mucus hostility.

Anyway, we eventually had a bouncing little boy, Andrew, nine months old now and gigantic. I keep taking the zinc in the hope that it will one day happen again. It has all been worth it.

· *Weight* ·

Weight loss in men has already been touched upon. For women, both excess and insufficient weight can be a cause of infertility. There is a range of weights for any given height which are considered healthy. If your weight (see chart on the next page) is above or below that range, it may be the cause of fertility problems.

Overweight women

Women who are overweight may have irregular menstrual cycles, have periods either very rarely or not at all, and fail to ovulate. Conventional treatment with anti-estrogens and gonadotropins (see page 41) is frequently unsuccessful in such women,[9] and it is thought that that excess weight may be responsible for polycystic ovary syndrome (PCOS), rather than a result of it.

A group of German doctors took 35 obese women who had been infertile for between five and six and a half years and encouraged them to take part in a weight-reducing plan which involved reducing their calorie intake and encouraging them to increase their physical activity. The scheme lasted for 14 to 32 weeks and the results were dramatic.

The women's Body Mass Index (BMI) weights at the start of the program were between 30.8 and 37.3 kg/m^2 (around 182 pounds 4 ounces to approximately 210 pounds for a woman of 5 foot 5 inches) and they each lost between 7.9 and 10.2 kg. (17 pounds 4 ounces to 22 pounds 4 ounces). Only seven did not show any improvement in their menstrual cycles and ten out of 35 conceived, eight of whom went on to have healthy babies (74.30 percent had

Weight	Kg																								
238 lbs	107	58	56	55	53	52	50	49	48	46	45	44	43	42	41	40	39	38	37	36	35	35	34	33	32
	106	57	56	54	53	51	50	48	47	46	45	44	42	41	40	39	38	38	37	36	35	34	33	33	32
	105	57	55	54	52	51	49	48	47	45	44	43	42	41	40	39	38	37	36	35	35	34	33	32	32
231 lbs	104	56	55	53	52	50	49	47	46	45	44	43	42	41	40	39	38	37	36	35	34	34	33	32	31
	103	56	54	53	51	50	48	47	46	45	43	42	41	40	39	38	37	36	36	35	34	33	33	32	31
	102	55	54	52	51	49	48	47	45	44	43	42	41	40	39	38	37	36	35	34	34	33	32	31	31
224 lbs	101	55	53	52	50	49	47	46	45	44	43	42	40	39	38	38	37	36	35	34	33	33	32	31	**30**
	100	54	53	51	50	48	47	46	44	43	42	41	40	39	38	37	36	35	35	34	33	32	32	31	**30**
	99	54	52	51	49	48	46	45	44	43	42	41	40	39	38	37	36	35	34	33	33	32	31	31	**30**
217 lbs	98	53	51	50	49	47	46	45	44	42	41	40	39	38	37	36	36	35	34	33	33	32	31	**30**	**30**
	97	52	51	49	48	47	46	44	43	42	41	40	39	38	37	36	35	34	34	33	32	31	31	**30**	29
	96	52	50	49	48	46	45	44	43	42	40	39	38	37	36	35	34	33	33	32	31	**30**	**30**	29	
210 lbs	95	51	50	48	47	46	45	43	42	41	40	39	38	37	36	35	34	33	33	32	31	31	**30**	**29**	29
	94	51	49	48	47	45	44	43	42	41	40	39	38	37	36	35	34	33	33	32	31	**30**	**30**	29	28
	93	50	49	47	46	45	44	42	41	40	39	38	37	36	35	34	33	34	33	32	31	31	**30**	**29**	28
203 lbs	92	50	48	47	46	44	43	42	41	40	39	38	37	36	35	34	33	33	32	31	**30**	**30**	29	28	28
	91	49	48	46	45	44	43	42	40	39	38	37	36	36	35	34	33	32	31	31	**30**	29	29	28	27
	90	49	47	46	45	43	42	41	40	39	38	37	36	35	34	33	33	32	31	**30**	**30**	29	28	28	27
196 lbs	89	48	47	45	44	43	42	41	40	39	38	37	36	35	34	33	32	31	**30**	29	29	28	27	27	
	88	48	46	45	44	42	41	40	39	38	37	36	35	34	34	33	32	31	**30**	**30**	29	28	28	27	27
	87	47	46	44	43	42	41	40	39	38	37	36	35	34	34	33	32	31	**30**	29	29	28	27	27	26
	86	46	45	44	43	41	40	39	38	37	36	35	34	34	33	32	31	**30**	**30**	29	28	28	27	27	26
189 lbs	85	46	45	43	42	41	40	39	38	37	36	35	34	33	32	32	31	**30**	29	29	28	27	27	26	26
	84	45	44	43	42	41	39	38	37	36	35	34	33	32	31	**30**	**30**	29	28	28	27	27	26		25
	83	45	44	42	41	40	39	38	37	36	35	34	33	32	31	**30**	29	29	28	27	27	26	26	25	
182 lbs	82	44	43	42	41	40	38	37	36	35	34	33	32	31	**30**	**30**	29	28	28	27	26	26	25	25	
	81	44	43	41	40	39	38	37	36	35	34	33	32	31	**30**	29	29	28	27	27	26	26	25	24	
	80	43	42	41	40	39	38	37	36	35	34	33	32	31	**30**	29	28	28	27	26	26	25	25	24	
175 lbs	79	43	41	40	39	38	37	36	35	34	33	32	32	31	**30**	29	29	28	27	27	26	26	25	24	24
	78	42	41	40	39	38	37	36	35	34	33	32	31	**30**	29	29	28	27	26	26	25	25	24	24	
	77	42	40	39	38	37	36	35	34	33	32	32	31	**30**	29	29	28	27	27	26	25	25	24	24	23
168 lbs	76	41	40	39	38	37	36	35	34	33	32	31	**30**	**30**	29	28	28	27	26	25	25	24	23	23	
	75	41	39	38	37	36	35	34	33	32	32	31	**30**	29	29	28	27	26	25	25	24	23	23		
	74	40	39	38	37	36	35	34	33	32	31	**30**	**30**	29	28	28	27	26	26	25	24	24	23	23	22
161 lbs	73	39	38	37	36	35	34	33	32	32	31	**30**	29	29	28	27	27	26	25	25	24	24	23	23	22
	72	39	38	37	36	35	34	33	32	31	**30**	**30**	29	28	27	27	26	25	24	24	23	23	22	22	
	71	38	37	36	35	34	33	32	32	31	**30**	29	28	28	27	26	26	25	25	24	23	23	22	22	21
154 lbs	70	38	37	36	35	34	33	32	31	**30**	29	28	28	27	27	26	25	25	24	24	23	23	22	22	21
	69	37	36	35	34	33	32	32	31	**30**	29	28	28	27	26	26	25	24	24	23	23	22	22	21	21
	68	37	36	35	34	33	32	31	**30**	29	28	28	27	27	26	25	25	24	24	23	22	22	21	21	21
147 lbs	67	36	35	34	33	32	31	31	**30**	29	28	28	27	26	26	25	24	24	23	23	22	22	21	20	20
	66	36	35	34	33	32	31	**30**	29	29	28	27	26	26	25	25	24	23	23	22	22	21	21	20	20
	65	35	34	33	32	31	**30**	**30**	29	28	27	27	26	25	25	24	24	23	22	22	21	21	20	20	
140 lbs	64	35	34	33	32	31	**30**	29	28	28	27	26	26	25	24	24	23	23	22	22	21	21	20	20	19
	63	34	33	32	31	**30**	**30**	29	28	27	27	26	25	25	24	23	23	22	22	21	21	20	20	19	19
	62	34	33	32	31	**30**	29	28	28	27	26	25	25	24	24	23	22	22	21	21	20	20	19	19	
133 lbs	61	33	32	31	**30**	29	29	28	27	26	26	25	24	24	23	23	22	22	21	21	20	20	19	19	**18**
	60	32	32	31	**30**	29	28	27	27	26	25	25	24	23	23	22	22	21	21	20	20	19	19	19	**18**
	59	32	31	**30**	29	28	28	27	26	26	25	24	24	23	23	22	22	21	20	20	19	19	19	**18**	**18**
126 lbs	58	31	**30**	**30**	29	28	27	26	26	25	24	24	23	23	22	22	21	20	20	19	19	**18**	**18**	18	
	57	31	**30**	29	28	27	27	26	25	24	23	23	22	22	21	21	20	20	19	19	**18**	**18**	**18**	17	
	56	**30**	29	29	28	27	26	26	25	24	24	23	22	22	21	21	20	19	19	**18**	**18**	**18**	17	17	
119 lbs	55	**30**	29	28	27	27	26	25	24	24	23	23	22	21	21	20	20	19	19	19	**18**	**18**	17	17	17
	54	29	28	28	27	26	26	25	24	24	23	22	22	21	21	20	20	19	19	**18**	**18**	17	17	17	16
	53	29	28	27	26	26	25	24	24	23	22	22	21	21	20	19	19	**18**	**18**	**18**	17	17	16	16	
112 lbs	52	**28**	27	27	26	25	24	24	23	23	22	21	21	20	20	19	19	**18**	**18**	**18**	17	17	16	16	16
	51	**28**	27	26	25	25	24	23	23	22	21	20	20	20	19	19	**18**	**18**	**18**	17	17	16	16	16	
	50	**27**	26	26	25	24	23	23	22	22	21	21	20	20	19	19	**18**	17	17	17	16	16	16	15	15
105 lbs	49	**26**	**26**	25	24	24	23	22	22	21	21	20	20	19	19	**18**	**18**	17	17	17	16	16	15	15	15
	48	**26**	25	24	24	23	23	22	21	21	20	20	19	19	**18**	**18**	17	17	17	16	16	15	15	14	
	47	25	25	24	23	23	22	21	21	20	20	19	19	**18**	**18**	17	17	16	16	16	15	15	15	14	
98 lbs	46	25	24	23	23	22	22	21	20	20	19	19	**18**	**18**	**18**	17	17	16	16	16	15	15	14	14	
	45	24	24	23	22	22	21	20	20	19	19	**18**	**18**	**18**	17	17	16	16	15	15	15	14	14		
	44	24	23	22	22	21	21	20	20	19	19	**18**	**18**	17	17	16	16	16	15	15	14	14	14	13	
	43	23	23	22	21	21	20	19	19	**18**	**18**	17	17	16	16	16	15	15	14	14	14	13	13		
91 lbs	42	23	22	21	21	20	20	19	19	**18**	**18**	17	17	16	16	15	15	15	14	14	14	13	13	13	
	41	22	22	21	20	20	19	19	**18**	**18**	17	17	16	16	16	15	15	14	14	14	13	13	13	12	
	40	22	21	20	20	19	19	**18**	**18**	17	17	16	16	16	15	15	14	14	14	13	13	13	12	12	

| | | 4'6" | 7" | 8" | 9" | 10" | 11" | 5'0" | 1" | 2" | 3" | 4" | 5' | 6" | 7" | 8" | 9" | 10" | 11" | 6'0" | | | | | Height |
| | | 1.13 | 1.38 | 1.40 | 1.42 | 1.44 | 1.46 | 1.48 | 1.50 | 1.52 | 1.54 | 1.56 | 1.58 | 1.60 | 1.62 | 1.64 | 1.66 | 1.68 | 1.70 | 1.72 | 1.74 | 1.76 | 1.78 | 1.80 | 1.82 m |

BODY MASS INDEX CHART
The middle band of weight/height ratios is ideal for pregnancy.

primary infertility, 25.7 percent secondary infertility). The others returned to more regular menstrual bleeding patterns, ovulation or normalization of luteal phase insufficiency.

Other benefits included a reduction in blood glucose, insulin, androstenedionel dihydrotestosterone and estradiol concentrations. The authors speculate that the PCOS may be caused by obesity and a specific insulin sensitivity of ovarian tissue (perhaps genetically determined), so that excess weight and consequent high insulin levels in the blood actively lead to menstrual irregularity, infertility and, after a time of chronic anovulation, to PCOS. They mention that other authors[10] see PCOS not as a specific clinical disease but as a non-specific ovarian response to the state of chronic anovulation of any cause. In other words, obesity causes the anovulation and raised levels of androgens which lead to excessive body hair, instead of the other way round. The doctors considered the amount of weight loss necessary to bring about these changes was 3.4 to 5.6 kg, which is relatively little.

Weight loss is, of course, not necessarily easy to achieve. It can be helpful to attend a group that supports people who are trying to lose weight. You may find that there is a group led by your doctor or health center or run by a local clinic or health visitors. Commercial groups are also available.

Eating more healthily and exercising will also help regulate weight, but it is vital not to smoke instead of eating as smoking, too, can affect fertility adversely (see page 91).

Underweight women

It is possible to be too thin to conceive. Underweight women below BMI 19.1kg/m^2 (see chart on page 85) may be so short of nutrition that they fail to ovulate or menstruate. They may be poorly nourished for a number of reasons, including eating poorly and dieting. It could be due to a combination of factors—a very pressured lifestyle may mean eating only snacks, drinking lots of coffee, and perhaps smoking, too. This can make you wonderfully slim but do little for your fertility.

Eating well, and avoiding the pitfalls already mentioned, is likely to restore ovulation in women whose menstrual irregularities are due to being underweight, and they are likely to feel better too. In this situation, taking a good multivitamin and other supplements is to be recommended.

It is interesting to note that women who are or have been anorexic and those who are vegetarians are, for different reasons, likely to be deficient in zinc, a mineral that is essential for reproductive function. Anorexics and those who are underweight can be low in zinc because they eat very little, although some specialists believe that anorexia is caused by zinc deficiency rather than the other way around. Such people will also often fail to ovulate because they are so undernourished. Vegetarians may also be zinc deficient, partly because they eat fewer foods that contain zinc—meat, poultry and shellfish being good sources—and also because phytic acid within plant fiber, especially wheat, combines with zinc to form insoluble compounds which are excreted and so not absorbed (see page 75).

Underweight women who conceive without ovulation induction are three times more likely than average to have a baby that is small for its gestational age, and those underweight women who become pregnant only after ovulation has been artificially stimulated are at even greater risk of having a low birth-weight baby, with the attendant health risks to the baby that are involved.[11]

If you are underweight, you should have three nutrient-rich meals a day. It is particularly important to eat breakfast. Breakfast cereals are fortified with B vitamins, folic acid and iron, and one study found that mothers who ate breakfast cereal were more likely to have healthy-sized babies.[12] You should aim to get your weight so that it registers BMI 20–25.

Excessive exercise can affect ovulation and sperm count—while being fit is excellent, over-training can result in a loss of periods and ovulation or a drop in testosterone levels. According to Sarah Brewer in *Planning a Baby?*, men who trained more than four days a week had a dramatically lowered sperm count. She describes a trial involving men who normally trained two or three times a week. When they doubled the amount they trained, their sperm concentrations dropped by 43 percent and remained low or lower, down to 52 percent less, for three months, and the number of immature and nonviable sperm they produced increased as well.

Vigorous exercise for at least 20 minutes, three times a week, is strongly recommended. Several women in a National Childbirth Trust article on running during pregnancy, considered that taking up running had helped them to overcome secondary infertility.[13] If you do much more than this consider whether you are doing too much and becoming too fit as far as your fertility is concerned.

· *Drugs* ·

Drugs, other than fertility enhancing drugs, can adversely affect your fertility. It is worth considering what you are consuming apart from food. You may not have thought that any of the drugs you take, either prescribed, over-the-counter or street drugs, could affect fertility. This category also includes smoking (see page 91) and alcohol (see page 69), both of which are known to decrease fertility.

Women and drugs

You should think about every drug you take. The fact that there is no proven link between a particular drug and infertility does not mean that it does not exist, or that it might not affect your fertility.

You should always let your doctor know that you are trying to conceive whenever drugs are prescribed for you. This also applies to the dentist, either before accepting pain-killing injections or a dental X ray, or if you have an X ray for any other reason. Some treatments may be reviewed if there is a possibility that you may be pregnant. Some drugs, some antibiotics for example, can have detrimental effects on a baby and others, such as danazol, prescribed for endometriosis, require you to stop taking them for some time (three months in the case of danazol) before attempting to conceive. You should remind the doctor every time and not depend on him or her to remember your situation as mistakes can easily be made. Drugs that can cause menstrual irregularities include drugs for migraine, nausea and vomiting, travel sickness, chemotherapy, anti-cancer drugs, and cortisone.

Over-the-counter drugs

Think about what you take in the way of over-the-counter medications. Nonsteroidal anti-inflammatories (NSAIDs) such as aspirin have been shown to delay follicular rupture in women and inhibit ovulation in rabbits.[14]

You should be particularly careful about what you take from around the time of ovulation until your period. Acetaminophen is generally considered safer than aspirin during pregnancy, especially in the first three months of pregnancy. Check the labels on proprietary painkillers; some contain aspirin. Others contain codeine, which has been linked with birth defects.[15]

Gels, creams, ointments, suppositories, and vaginal deodorants should be used with caution or not at all.

Some antihistamines and anti-inflammatories can have the effect of drying up cervical secretions.

Street drugs

Marijuana can cause menstrual-cycle irregularities and it also affects cell division. It should not be taken pre-conceptually or in pregnancy, as it can affect fetal growth and result in low birth-weight babies.

Amphetamines, barbiturates, and cocaine can all cause miscarriage or premature birth and/or birth defects, and stillbirth.

Heroin, methadone, LSD, PCP, solvents and glue can all cause miscarriage or fetal abnormalities or behavioral abnormalities in babies born to mothers who take them.

Anyone taking recreational drugs is strongly recommended to stop when trying to conceive or while pregnant.

For help in stopping drugs or alcohol see Useful Addresses.

Antidepressants

Researchers have discovered a link between women who have had clinical depression and a risk of ovulatory infertility. Doubts have been expressed as to whether antidepressants cause infertility problems or whether infertility has resulted in depression. Although it is still not clear whether drugs or depression are responsible for the infertility, one study suggests that half the women had depression before they started trying to conceive.

If you are taking antidepressants, discuss your situation with your doctor and see if he or she can provide you with some other kind of help, such as counseling. The organizations mentioned in the Useful Addresses section (National Institute for Alcohol and Drug Information, National Institute on Drug Abuse, and the Do It Now Foundation) may be able to offer support.

You may also find practicing relaxation techniques, hypnotherapy, medical herbalism, or reflexology helpful.

Men and drugs

Remember that smoking and alcohol (see pages 91 and 69) come into this category.

Remind your doctor that you are trying for a baby before drugs are prescribed, as fewer prescription drugs are thought to affect fertility in men than in women, but drugs taken to treat cancer may affect sperm. Tranquilizers and drugs taken to lower blood pressure can reduce your sex drive.

Over-the-counter drugs

Little is known about the adverse affects that these might have on male fertility, but is important to be cautious, particularly about creams and ointments.

Street drugs

As for women.

Anabolic steroids

Many men do not realize that taking anabolic steroids in order to enhance body-building can cause sterility. Taking large doses leads to a reduction in spermatogenesis and in the size of testicles.

Among other effects, it can induce hypergonadotropic hypogonadism and mean that no sperm are produced at all. In fact, the drugs have been considered for use as male contraceptives.

Detailed case histories[16] show how effective anabolic steroids are in causing azoospermia in men who have previously fathered children and make it clear that only stopping them completely will reverse the situation. It can take up to twelve months for sperm to return to normal, and in some cases the ill effects may last as long as three years.[17]

There is no evidence that human chorionic gonadotropins will have any protective effect.

In some cases, men taking health drinks offered by their gym are unaware that they are taking anabolic steroids.

Other side effects include alterations in lipid concentrations, liver disease, jaundice, liver tumors, developing breasts, mood changes, reduction in sex drive, dependence, withdrawal effects, and cancer of the prostate gland.

· *Smoking* ·

Smoking has been described as the foremost reproductive poison of the twentieth century[18] and there can be little doubt that it reduces fertility.[19] A review of 48 studies of the effect of smoking showed that smoking by women clearly reduced their chances of conceiving, and that the effect was dose-dependent, i.e. the more they smoked the less likely they were to conceive. In one study[20] women who smoked fewer than 20 cigarettes a day were 25 percent less fertile than nonsmokers, and those who smoked more than 20 a day were 43 percent less likely to conceive. Although different studies produce slightly different results, there can be no doubt that smoking in women can considerably delay conception. It also has a drastic effect on the ability to maintain a pregnancy. In a large study of 108 smokers and 542 nonsmokers who were undergoing IVF and GIFT[21] the authors found that there was a similar fertilization rate between both groups, but a reduction in clinical pregnancy rate (8 percent versus 22 percent) and an increase in the miscarriage rate between smokers and nonsmokers (55 percent versus 20 percent). Caffeine intake, age and smoking in the male partner were not taken into consideration, but nonetheless, the difference that smoking or not smoking makes seems considerable.

There is also a lot of evidence, based on studies of a total of 100,000 women, which suggests that miscarriage following natural conception is more likely in smokers, with the likelihood increasing the more that the women smoked.

It is thought that smoking has such detrimental effects on conception and the developing embryo because tobacco smoke contains a complex mixture of toxins which affect sperm production, tubal motility, embryo division, blastocyst (fertilized egg at the time of implantation) formation, growth of the inner cell mass, and implantation. In animal studies cigarette smoke has been shown to affect various levels of reproductive function, including the hypothalamic-pituitary axis, testes, ovaries, and uterus. In a woman, it reduces circulating levels of estrogen; those who smoke more than 20 a day have menopause on average two years earlier than nonsmokers, which may be due to accelerated egg depletion.

Less conclusive evidence shows that smoking impairs men's fertility, although there are studies which show this, and it seems likely that if it can affect sperm production, smoking can damage male fertility, too. Moreover, recent evidence shows that passive smoking can affect a woman's ovaries.

Of course, smoking should not be seen in isolation. In addition to the well-known risk of causing lung cancer, it can have other less well-known side effects. These include coronary heart disease, chronic bronchitis and emphysema, stroke, other atherosclerotic peripheral vascular disease, and osteoporosis.

In pregnancy, women who smoke have a 27 percent higher chance of miscarrying, are twice as likely to go into premature labor, have an enhanced chance of ectopic pregnancy and of having placenta praevia (where the placenta covers the cervix partially or totally, preventing a vaginal birth), or placenta abruptio (where the placenta peels away before the birth, causing shock, hemorrhage, and risking the baby's life).

Even if pregnancy goes to full term, the baby of a mother who has smoked through pregnancy is still very disadvantaged. It is 33 percent more likely than babies of nonsmokers to be still-born or die shortly after birth. It will on average be 7 ounces lighter and be at risk from sudden infant death syndrome (crib death). If either parent smokes after the baby's birth, this greatly increases the risk that the baby will suffer from ill health, in particular from asthma and ear infections, and will be admitted to the hospital with health problems.

All in all, it is quite clear that couples trying to conceive, especially those experiencing difficulties, should stop smoking. However, this is notoriously difficult, even when people are convinced of the value of doing it, and it may take considerable effort. One study showed that even when given specific advice and encouragement to stop during an IVF cycle, only 20 percent of women managed to do it. It is undeniably hard, but not impossible. Some of the alternative therapies such as acupuncture and hypnotherapy can definitely help.

Your health center or hospital should be able to put you in touch with a support group to help you stop smoking. If possible, find someone, either a health professional or a friend, who will offer you one-on-one support, and encourage you along the way. The key thing is really wanting to stop: many women with fertility problems would do anything to have a baby. Even if your fertility problems are not directly connected to smoking, it cannot improve your chances of conceiving or your baby's chance of survival. Don't give up if you don't succeed at once, but persist and get more help. You can contact Nicotine Anonymous for quitting support (see Useful Addresses). Nicotine Anonymous is a twelve-step organization dedicated to combating nicotine addiction.

It really is important for both of you to stop smoking, even if the male partner seems to have super-sperm, partly because of the risks of passive smoking, and also because it has been shown that there is an increased risk of cancer among people whose fathers were smokers. You need to support each other in this—perhaps exercise together more and break the smoking routine.

· *Chemicals (estrogens and toxins)* ·

Estrogens

Although the case is not clear-cut, concern has been growing about an overall decrease in sperm levels, increases in testicular cancer and the number of babies being born with undescended testes, and deformity or abnormality of the penis. The case for and against estrogens has been debated intensely, but there is certainly cause for concern. Speculation revolves around the question of whether the estrogens that we consume unwittingly are the cause, either because what pregnant women eat affects male babies before birth or because they are consumed after birth, and have a feminizing effect on boys and men then.

Between 1945 and 1971 several million women who were experiencing a threatened miscarriage during pregnancy were given diethylstilbestrol (DES), a synthetic estrogen, to preserve their pregnancies. At the time no one knew that this could have serious effects upon their unborn children, causing cancer and sterility in girls and increasing the levels of cryptorchism (undescended testes) and hypospadias (a defect in the penis) and decreased semen volume and sperm counts in later life in boys.

Although DES has been banned from use, there are several other ways in which we are exposed to estrogens, both before birth and in everyday life. Some are within our power to limit, others are not.

It is thought that dietary changes may be responsible for our ingesting extra estrogen. Women in particular on low-fiber diets may not effectively excrete the estrogens they take in, so that they are recirculated within the body. Increased body fat can lead to higher levels of estrogen within the body because it can convert other steroids into estrogens and obesity can decrease the level of sex hormone-binding globulin (SHBG) to which estrogens are naturally bonded. Low levels of SHBG mean that the estrogen has a more powerful effect on the body.

Synthetic estrogens, such as are found in the pill, can be

found in drinking water. They are particularly potent because they do not bond to SHBG.

Anabolic estrogens were used in the agricultural treatment of livestock between the 1950s and 1970s although their use has been banned in Europe since 1981. Cow's milk is naturally high in estrogens as most dairy cows are pregnant while producing milk.

Many food plants contain weak estrogens, such as soy, which is increasingly used as a meat substitute, being one of the richest sources. However, plant estrogens may increase the amount of SHBG, thus reducing the potency of endogenous estrogens.

Perhaps the most contentious source of estrogen, and an area in which we have least individual control, is that of environmental chemicals. Over 50,000 artificial chemicals have been developed since the 1930s. Many of these, known as organochlorines, are weakly estrogenic but do not biodegrade easily, and are accumulating in the food chain and within our bodies. Although some of these, such as polychlorinated biphenyls (PCBs) and dichlorodiphenyltrichloroethane (DDT), have now been banned, they are still present in the atmosphere—as are those produced by the internal combustion engine.

Debate continues as to whether in fact sperm counts are dropping generally, but it would seem to make sense on current advice to:

eat organic food
limit your intake of dairy products and fats
drink bottled water
eat a moderately high-fiber diet
maintain or achieve reasonable weight
limit the amount of soy you eat
use lead-free gasoline

Insecticides and pesticides

There is no doubt that pesticides, insecticides, and herbicides can damage human fertility. There are examples of serious and permanent infertility caused by agricultural pesticides. In Costa Rica, 1500 men—a huge number—became sterile as a result of exposure to a toxic nematicide which was used to treat bananas in large commercial plantations.[22]

In Europe a study found that fruit growers who used pesticides on their trees had a very substantially reduced fertility—28 percent of those who had high levels of exposure to pesticides had sought help because of the couples" problems in failing to become pregnant. Their chances of conception were much greater out of the spraying season (March to November).[23]

Other reports of couples seeking AID (artificial insemination by donor) indicate higher numbers among men whose jobs involve long-term exposure to pesticides and insecticides.[24]

It is not only male fertility that may be affected by pesticide use—it can also be responsible for pregnancy complications, such as miscarriage, intrauterine growth retardation, fetal abnormalities, and stillbirth.[25]

It is important to be aware that all pesticides are potentially damaging—they are intended to kill, after all—and not just the ones to which people are exposed while at work. Anyone who has fertility problems, is trying to conceive, or is pregnant should be particularly aware of, and avoid contact with, things like woodworm killer, wood preservatives, paints and sprays, insecticides, plant fungicides, and head-lice treatments (lindane, for example, has been banned in fourteen countries).

Toxins

It may pay to be very suspicious of anything that smells particularly strongly and be aware of how it affects you. Some treatments and chemicals do provide warning signs by causing headaches and other immediate symptoms. It is best to avoid chemicals as far as possible, including air fresheners, hair dyes, strong cleansing agents, bleaches, strong perfumes, and aftershaves. Anecdotal evidence has linked some causes of infertility with air fresheners. A drop of essential oil of thyme or pine oil, in water is as antiseptic as commercial air fresheners.

If you have to use paints or pesticides, make sure that there is a good ventilator and use an effective mask which will filter out the fumes.

Occupational hazards

If you are aware that you are exposed to chemicals at work, you may be faced with difficult decisions. Clearly, it is important that any health and safety regulations are followed, but it is possible that these may not be adequate. Talk to your employer about your concerns and see if any further protection is available; you may have to explain why you are worried. There may be steps that you can take yourself to avoid additional exposure, and you can contact the Center for Nuclear and Toxic Waste Management, which provides World Wide Web links to academic reports, government sites, and citizens' action groups on toxic chemicals (see Useful Addresses). If it turns out that there is no way of reducing your exposure, even if only for a few months, you may have to think about changing your job.

- Be aware of household chemicals and minimize their use—use plant alternatives where possible.
- Use pesticides only when absolutely essential—use alternatives such as pyrethrum liquid, on plants.
- Wear a good air-filter mask when using chemicals, solvents, paint, preservatives.
- Don't use strong-smelling perfumes, after-shaves or deodorants.
- Don't use air-fresheners.
- Be aware of chemicals in your workplace; follow health and safety regulations or manufacturer's advice scrupulously.
- Wear a mask at work when appropriate.
- If you think that work hazards are causing your fertility problems, discuss it with your employer or personnel officer.
- If chemicals remain unavoidable and you are unable to change how you work, consider changing your job or occupation.

The following is a list of chemicals which have been identified by a WWF report on pesticides posing hazards to reproduction as having effects on reproduction and/or possible effects on reproductive hormones.

2, 4-DB	HCB
2, 4-D and 2, 4, 5-T	heptachlor
alachlor	lindane (head-lice treatment)
aminotriazole	linuron
amitraz	methomyl
benomyl	methoxychlor
B—HCH	metribuzin
bromoxynil and ioxynil	mirex
carbaryl	molinate
carbendazim	nitrofen
carbofuran	organophosphates
chlordane	pentachlorophenol
chlordecone	permethrin
chlordimeform	phenothrin
conazole fungicides	phenylphenol
DBCP	procymidone
DDT	pyrethroids
dicofol	quizalofop-ethyl
dieldrin	TBT
dinoseb	toxaphene
dioxin	trans-nonachlor
dithiocarbamates	triazine herbicides
EDB	trifluralin
endosulfan	triforine
fenarimolfentin acetate	vinvlozolin
fluazifop—butyl	

The report is available from:

World Wildlife Fund
1250 24th Street NW
Washington, DC 20037
Tel: 800-CALL-WWF
Web site: www.worldwildlife.org

· *Everyday considerations* ·

Men

Heat

It has long been established that the testes hang from the body, rather than being contained within it, because sperm can only be produced at a temperature of 32 °C. (89°F), which is five degrees below normal body temperature. Maintaining this temperature is crucial. If it is raised for any reason, sperm counts drop.

There are a number of reasons why testicular temperature may be raised. First, clothing: tight underpants or jeans can keep testicles close to the body so that they are unable to dangle and air cannot circulate around them. Wearing looser pants and boxer shorts can significantly improve fertility. One study of sperm donors involved persuading them to alternate boxer shorts with tight underwear for three months and vice versa for a total of twelve months. Dramatic effects were recorded: sperm volume, density, motility, and total numbers were all reduced by between 7 percent to 21 percent while the men were wearing tight underwear. Although they would probably still have been fertile, choice of underpants could make the difference between subfertility and fertility in men. Improvements began to be noticed within two weeks of wearing the boxer shorts, which was sooner than might have been expected.

Interestingly, electricity generated by polyester underwear is able to create an electrostatic field which is able to not only reduce sperm count significantly but also cause testicular degeneration. In fact, a combination of polyester and tight underwear in the form of a polyester jockstrap was so effective at reducing sperm production that it could be used as a method of contraception, having totally stopped spermogenesis in 14 volunteers after 140 days of wearing the sling.

Cotton underwear generate no electrical charge, so wearing cotton boxer shorts together with loose-fitting pants provides the best way of maintaining testicles at the right temperature.

Daily hot baths of 43–45°C (109–113°F), or more, lasting half an hour, can lower sperm count, so it would be best to keep the bath temperature down. For the same reason also avoid saunas.

Electric blankets should be avoided. There is anecdotal evidence that they can cause fertility problems and it seems very probable, given that heat reduces male fertility.

A French study which questioned couples about the time it took them to become pregnant uncovered the fact that men driving for more than three hours a day led to a delay in their patients becoming pregnant. Driving raises testicular temperature in a similar way to wearing tight clothing. It is also recognized that other occupations which involve exposure to heat such as welding and deep sea diving, can have an adverse effect on male fertility.

Occupation

People's jobs are too varied to consider in specific detail, but it may be useful to look critically at what your job involves, bearing in mind the known factors which have the potential to reduce fertility. For example:

- Atmosphere—does your work expose you to gases or fumes which you inhale? Anesthetists, for example, are said to have reduced fertility and are more likely to father girls.
- Radiation—does your work involve radiation, for example X rays or airport security devices?
- Heat (see above.)
- Chemicals—do you handle chemicals, sprays or solvents, or work with substances such as insecticides, pesticides, and herbicides that are designed to kill? (See pages 95–98.)
- Does any chemically treated substance in your workplace give you symptoms when, or after, you come into contact with it? It will probably have a strong smell; it could be a new office building, chemicals in carpets, paints, varnishes, etc. Your job may involve supplying such products.
- Diet—do you eat poorly or little while at work, or smoke or drink alcohol?
- Clothes—do you wear a uniform or work clothes which restrict your testicles?

- Drink—what do you drink and where does it come from? Do you drink enough or are you dehydrated?
- Exercise—some jobs involve small, moderate, or even large amounts of exercise, but if you are sitting down all day you should be getting some exercise when you are not working.
- Stress—do you find your work stressful? (See below.)

There is considerable evidence to show that stress can play a part in reducing male fertility.[26] For example, just the knowledge that a man has to produce a sperm sample for IVF treatment has been shown to reduce normal sperm qualities significantly, so that concentration, total count, morphology, and sperm motility are all reduced by the stress of the experience.

It has also been shown[27] that when semen samples from men under stress were compared with those who were not, the samples from the stressed group were decreased in volume and had a lower rate of normal morphology. Animal experiments have proved that fertility can be reduced in male monkeys by subjecting them to stress.[28]

If you are finding your job stressful, you must either change it or find ways of coping with it. Only you can decide whether you can make a change, either to a different job within the same field or by moving into a different sphere altogether, perhaps by retraining or doing something financially less rewarding but more satisfying and less stressful. If you feel that you have no choice, you may be helped by learning and practicing relaxation techniques (see pages 164–66) or by trying one of the alternative therapies that are particularly good at helping people deal with stress, for example herbal medicine, hypnotherapy, and reflexology.

Women

Occupations

It is possible that your work environment may be affecting you adversely too. Although the effect of atmospheric toxins on women is less well documented than that for men, it is still possible for your reproductive health to be damaged by your working conditions. Observe the effects your work or workplace are having on you, especially if you work in an atmosphere that is strong-smelling or where there are fumes, for example at a dry cleaners, hairdresser's, or a factory where paints, solvents, or textile dyes are used, if you sit close to a photocopying machine, or work in an office which is new or has new furnishings and fittings that smell strongly. You might become suspicious if you get headaches or feel ill only when you are at work or just after you leave, and not when you are not there. Excessively noisy workplaces have been found to cause delayed conception, hormonal disturbances, and infertility. Exposure to lead, cadmium, and mercury can have a similar effect.[29]

It is particularly difficult when colleagues become pregnant and you do not (see Chapter 4), but you should not assume that your work environment cannot be the cause of the problem if other women there are able to become pregnant. Everyone reacts individually, they may simply have a stronger constitution or there may be other factors which make them able to conceive.

Work-related stress could have a bearing on your difficulties. Women can be under such pressure that their bodies seem to consider that they are unable to cope with pregnancy on top of everything else. Many women become pregnant after reducing their working hours or otherwise lessening pressure at work.

When you are very involved with a job, it can be extremely difficult to stand back and see whether the demands it makes or the demands you make of yourself are excessive. You may be throwing yourself into your job in order to forget about your fertility problems, or the job itself may require so much of you that you have little time or energy left for anything else. No one is absolutely indispensable. Remember too that, to a varying degree, every woman has some time off if she does become pregnant and give birth. You may need to consider whether your work is putting you under such pressure that it may be making conception harder, and take steps to lessen the load if you are doing too much.

Alternatively, you may enjoy it so much that it makes you ambivalent about becoming pregnant. It is clear that to some extent fertility is under subconscious control; perhaps you should examine your motivations and be honest with yourself about any blocks or barriers, physical or mental, that you may feel are in your way.

· *Francesca* ·

We started trying for a baby three years ago. I had been on the pill for three years and so stopped and tried to do everything right, like checking my rubella immunity. Although I had no problems with the pill while I was on it, and on the two previous occasions that I had taken it, when I stopped it this time my periods started coming every 14 days and then I had a 50-day interval.

I went to my GP, who did a blood test. She said that my luteinizing hormone levels were raised; another test showed low levels and it did not look promising. She wondered whether I might have polycystic ovary syndrome. At the same time she referred my husband for a sperm count, which came back as being relatively normal.

My doctor put me on Clomid, which did make me ovulate but I did not get pregnant. The drug gave me hot flashes and meant that I did not have proper night vision. My vision failed once while I was driving which was very frightening.

My GP then referred me to our local hospital, but it turned out that the appointment would not be for nine months, which I found very frustrating. I hated being out of control and the feeling that nothing was happening. The only thing that I felt I could do to help myself was make temperature charts. I joined CHILD [Note: This is a fertility organization in the UK; for American resources see Useful Addresses] and consequently got in touch with an alternative health practitioner that they recommend. I still had to wait quite a long time to see her, but when we finally did she assessed us both.

We had both had post-viral syndrome and as a consequence she found that our vitamin and mineral levels were 30 to 40 percent of what they should have been. She also thought that we were allergic to various foods, such as yeast, tomatoes, dairy products, chocolate, coffee, shrimp, and beef.

She put us on an exclusion diet for six weeks which involved eating little besides brown rice and raw vegetables, and suggested various vitamin and mineral supplements. After three weeks we both started to feel much better and after six weeks we were able to start introducing foods. We were all right on everything except beef and shrimp, which we could happily do without. Our vitamin levels started to rise. Then the practitioner sent my husband to a private clinic to have his sperm tested. The result came back saying the amount of sperm was negligible, which upset everything. My blood test showed that I should ovulate in about 21 days.

In the meantime we had an NHS appointment. I had two blood tests which showed that I was all right and when they checked my husband's sperm count it was OK. They upped my dose of Clomid to 100, even though tests showed that I was ovulating. I then had a laparoscopy and they managed to perforate my bladder. I got an infection and had to spend ten days in the hospital on antibiotics.

While we were on the vitamins and minerals it was costing around $60 a month, which was very little compared with having anything done privately, and it meant that I was doing something to help myself. Besides, it was making us feel better, so there were advantages even if I didn't become pregnant.

The doctor advised us to wait three months and then, at the end of December 1995, she said that our levels were absolutely right and that it would be all right to start trying. As it happened, although I didn't realize it at the time, I was already pregnant.

I carried on taking the vitamins throughout my pregnancy and eventually gave birth to 9 lb 1½ oz Matilda, who is now 21 weeks and absolutely fine.

· *Ovulation detection* ·

Many women with fertility problems will be all too aware of when they are or are not ovulating. Moreover, it is possible to buy ovulation kits or even a fertility computer to test daily urine samples to pinpoint, with the aid of reactive tests, the optimum days for conception just before ovulation takes place. However, using these regularly is quite expensive, mildly inconvenient, and can reduce spontaneity still further. They can be useful if you are not sure whether or not you are ovulating at all. However, it can also be very helpful to be able to recognize your bodily symptoms, so that you can be aware of ovulation and the indications that it is about to take place without the need for tests or even taking your temperature.

It may take a little while to get used to checking for signs of ovulation, but once learned, it can be very useful. It consists of observing the changes in cervical mucus, feeling for changes in the cervix, and becoming aware of any other signs of ovulation that may be unique to you. You may want to double-check with the thermometer or tests to begin with, but this should soon become unnecessary.

Start by feeling your cervix every day, perhaps beginning at the end of a period, although you don't need to wait until then before practicing.

Wash your hands thoroughly, leave your fingers wet, and then either squat or sit on the toilet, and insert one or two fingers into your vagina. Push them up as far as they will go. The cervix at the top of your vagina will feel like a firm smooth knob with a little indentation in the inside, this is the os, or opening. As your cycle progresses the position of your cervix and its shape will alter. The uterus is suspended by the pelvic ligaments. This means that it is mobile and rises and drops slightly in response to hormonal changes.

At the start of a cycle following a period the cervix can be felt low in the vagina. By the time ovulation occurs it will have risen by 2–3 centimeters to its highest point, where it may be hard to reach with your fingers. Following ovulation it descends again, becoming lowest just before a period.

The nature of your cervix will change too; at ovulation it will be softer and more accommodating. The os becomes looser, so that you may be able to insert a fingertip, and it will feel wet.

Cervical mucus, however, is the clearest sign of pre-ovulatory changes and will provide the best indication of when you are most likely to be fertile. Mucus which follows a period is fairly scanty, sticky, dry, opaque and pastelike. As ovulation approaches, the mucus becomes wetter and more slippery. It also becomes clearer and much more stretchy, so that you can stretch it between your fingers.

Mucus which is transparent, slippery, and stretchy—very similar to egg-white in appearance—is fertile mucus, which indicates that ovulation is likely to occur within the next few days. The maximum amount of mucus may be produced a day or two before ovulation, but any day in which it is present is a good day on which to have sex, because sperm are able to survive for around five days in fertile mucus. It is ideally structured to allow sperm to travel rapidly through it, being composed of loosely connected filaments which hold back defective sperm while allowing motile ones to slip through. (Cervical mucus will form a shape in water, whereas other secretions will dissolve.)

Following ovulation, the mucus will change quite quickly back to the sticky, opaque, non-elastic unfertile type. If you are trying to work out exactly when ovulation occurs purely by checking mucus, it may be possible only in retrospect. However, there are some other indicators, together with symptoms that are individual to you, which you will be aware of as you become accustomed to detecting ovulation in this way. They might include alteration in sex drive, vulval pressure, odd rashes, or spots or a change in the way you smell.

Other common signs of ovulation can include pain in the abdomen, maybe only on one side, which can last for a few minutes or several hours or longer. Some women experience breast pain or tingling at ovulation; a few have very light bleeding and some may notice the swelling and tenderness of a gland in the groin. The lump is about the size of a pea and is present on the same side as the ovary from which the egg is being discharged.

Temperature-taking

This is useful if you want confirmation that you are ovulating, but because a woman's temperature only rises after ovulation takes place, it is less satisfactory as a method of determining the best time to have sex, which is just before or at ovulation.

A woman's temperature on waking is raised by around 0.2° C (0.6–0.8°F) in the days following ovulation, because of the effects of the progesterone secreted by the corpus luteum. This higher temperature is maintained until the start of a period—or beyond if pregnancy has taken place. To make a basal body temperature (BBT) chart, take your temperature daily, either first thing in the morning before you get up, or at another set time, provided that in both cases you have had nothing to eat or drink beforehand. Buy a fertility thermometer or—perhaps easier—a battery-operated digital thermometer from a chemist. Using graph paper (or a ready-made chart) plot a chart with the days of the month along one axis and the possible range of temperature along the other. Take your temperature, then plot the result on the graph. Alternatively, keep a record of your temperature and plot in all the results at once, at the end of your cycle. If you join up the dots on the chart you will be able to see whether there is a consistently lower reading, followed by a steep rise and higher readings each month.

BBT charts are notoriously hard to interpret and temperature can be affected by illness, alcohol intake, medication, oversleeping, late nights, holidays, stress, traveling, etc. and therefore should not be relied on too heavily. For more information about BBT and other ways of determining ovulation, read *Taking Charge of Your Fertility* by Toni Weschler (see Further Reading).

ALTERNATIVE THERAPIES

· *Why try alternatives?* ·

There are many reasons for turning to alternative therapies to help with fertility problems, not least of which is that they can prove effective even in apparently hopeless cases.

If you decide to see a complementary therapist the matter is under your control. You can choose who to see and when to see them. You can refer yourself and become directly involved with your treatment. You will rarely have to wait long for an appointment and should be treated sympathetically. Should you not get along with the practitioner you can easily change to another one.

Most alternative therapies have a very long history, in some cases (acupuncture and herbal medicine, for example) dating back thousands of years. The treatment is holistic; you will find that greater attention is paid to all aspects of your medical history and past and present lifestyle, and you will be treated as a whole, with the emotional aspects of your situation taken into consideration as well as the physical. Both partners can be treated and other apparently unrelated problems, such as backache or headaches, may be treated successfully, too. The aim is to encourage your body to heal itself, and to that end a practitioner may be able to make objective suggestions about improving your diet, or increasing your strength or managing your time. You will be involved in helping to make any necessary changes. A good practitioner will be well aware of your emotional well-being and will be encouraging and supportive. You should see the same person consistently. He or she should provide a welcoming atmosphere which will give you the opportunity to air your problems one-on-one, and the treatment and discussion will promote your physical and mental relaxation.

The treatments, which may take place over several weeks or months, should enhance your well-being and increase your general health. Even a long course of treatment is likely to be cheaper than privately funded assisted conception, and treatments like these are safer than using drugs or techniques which have been developed comparatively recently, and may have undesirable long-term side effects. Drugs are often prescribed inappropriately and may also force one part of the body into action when overall you are not fit for parenthood. You may wish to use alternative treatments to complement assisted conception, or use them instead, or perhaps try the alternative therapy first, leaving ART in reserve. Either way, if you try any method of natural healing, you should find that it makes you feel better overall. As some of the stories in this book show, these therapies really can help overcome infertility, not only where it is unexplained but also in cases where people were told there was no hope.

· *Choosing a therapy and* ·
finding a therapist

You will probably find that one particular therapy will feel right for you. As you read through the following pages you may recognize something that appeals to you or find that you don't relish the idea of one type of treatment or another. Some people dislike the idea of needles, even the really fine ones used in acupuncture, or they may particularly enjoy the idea of lying back and relaxing while their feet are treated through reflexology.

Once you have decided which therapy you might like to try, find out whether anyone you know has used it. A word-of-mouth recommendation is the best way of selecting a good therapist, but you will also need to talk to them first. You may want to ask them whether they have expertise in treating people with your problem, how long they have been practicing, what their fees are, and so on. If you are unable to go on personal recommendation, contact the appropriate professional body for the therapy of your choice (see Useful

Addresses). They will send you a list of registered practitioners and should you contact one or more, talk to them on the phone or in person and get a feeling about whether you will be able to establish a rapport with them. Trust your instinct and, if you have any doubts, look for someone else. It is vital that you feel comfortable with the person you choose. Although several therapists may be able to work satisfactorily and successfully with you, you are putting yourself in a personal relationship with the one you choose and will probably see them quite often, so it is important that you like and trust them and are confident in their ability to help you.

Talk about fees and ask how many treatments you may require, or the minimum number they consider beneficial. If you will find it hard to pay, tell them, as they may reduce fees in cases of financial hardship. It can be daunting to ask all of this of someone you have never met before, especially if you have no experience of medical treatment other than via your GP, but a good practitioner will not mind and will be open to questioning. It is inadvisable to go ahead with someone who asks for money up front before you see them, anyone who tells you that you can't be feeling in a particular way or insists that you are responding to treatment in any way that you feel you are not. Be wary too of people who claim you must get your vitamins or minerals via their "prescription" (they may be receiving commission) or do not appear to be taking in what you say or concentrating solely on you.

If you are doubtful about your treatment or feel uneasy about what is being done, say so. If you are not happy with the response try someone or something else. There are plenty of excellent empathic alternative therapists who believe passionately in their work and find treating people, especially those with fertility problems, very rewarding.

· *Acupuncture* ·

Acupuncture is a complete system of medicine which was developed in China over 5,000 years ago. It is based on the theory that the body consists of two opposing parts, yin and yang. Yin is deep, cold, and female and yang is hot, stimulating, and male. In good health, yin and yang are perfectly balanced, but in illness the equilibrium is disturbed. It can be restored by acupuncture. It is thought that the organs of the body are joined by invisible pathways or meridians. Illness occurs when a meridian or energy pathway becomes obstructed, and pain and symptoms may be felt at any point along the meridian. An acupuncturist will insert very fine needles at the point where the meridian is blocked. This removes the blockage and allows the body's vital energy or Qi (pronounced chee) to flow freely along the meridians. Free-flowing Qi will keep blood circulating, warm the body, and fight disease. There are twelve main meridians and more than 365 acupuncture points, the recognized points where needles may be placed.

The philosophy evolved purely from observing people in ill health, at a time when doctors were not allowed to do surgery or perform postmortem examinations on bodies. Everything that doctors knew came from observing, questioning, and touching their patients. An acupuncturist will pay particular attention to your appearance, color, and smell as well as what you tell him or her about the way you feel. Your pulse will be especially informative; an experienced acupuncturist can detect fourteen different pulses in the wrist, each of which provides information about imbalances within the body.

Traditional Chinese medical diagnoses and descriptions of illness are completely different from Western ones. For example, a woman suffering from infertility might be diagnosed as being infertile due to "decline in essential energy." Treatment takes the form of inserting fine needles, a little thicker than a hair, at acupuncture points relevant to your particular problem. The needles stay in for half an hour or longer, while the acupuncturist checks your pulse periodically to see how you are responding. After about 40 minutes the needles are removed and you can go home. You may feel slightly giddy, light-headed, or tired on the way back. The needles usually hurt only briefly as they are inserted, although there may be a spell as treatment progresses when you are recovering and before you are better when they can hurt a bit more. In later sessions you may barely feel them.

Traditional Chinese acupuncturists would also make very specific recommendations about diet, recommending such foods as raspberries, strawberries, squid, and oysters to strengthen kidney yin in cases of deficiency, for example. It is interesting that suggested foods for infertility in both sexes may be those which contain a lot of zinc. It is also recognized that being over- or underweight may cause infertility. Reasons attributed to female infertility (such as jealousy) have less clear links, although there is little disputing the possibility of emotional causes.

Other adjuncts to acupuncture may include moxabustion, the burning of a stick of the dried herb mugwort close to various acupuncture points in order to warm them, and perhaps the application of press pins, needles a little bit like drawing-pins which can be taped over the points so that you can apply pressure yourself when at home. Chinese herbal medicine (see page 139) and acupressure techniques might also be prescribed.

Acupressure, also known as shiatsu, works in a similar way to acupuncture, but involves applying deep pressure rather than needles to the appropriate points. You can use it on yourself at any time once you know which points to press. If you are using acupressure on yourself, you will know when you have found the acupressure point because it will feel slightly tender and more sensitive than the surrounding areas. Although for fertility treatment you would need specialist guidance, it is possible to relieve everyday aches and pains yourself. (See Julian Kenyon's *Acupressure Techniques—A Self-Help Guide*.)

Bob Flaws in *Path of Pregnancy* recognizes that there may be particularly Western causes of female infertility, such as that which may result from D and C's, terminations, cesarean sections, appendectomies, and the use of suppressant drugs in the treatment of vaginitis, pelvic inflammatory disease, cystititis, and venereal disease. Male infertility can be treated through acupuncture and with the use of herbal formulas. It is important that these are prescribed individually, although ginseng and ginger appear to be helpful.

There is evidence from at least one trial of the effect that acupuncture can have in helping to overcome infertility.[1] This trial took 45 women who were infertile, 27 suffering from having very infrequent periods and 18 with luteal insufficiency, and matched them with another 45 with similar characteristics including length of time that they had been unable to conceive, weight, tubal patency, previous pregnancies, menstrual cycle, etc.

The first group were given acupuncture on the ear. (Like the feet and hands in reflexology, there are points on the ear which reflect different areas of the body, so a person can be treated via their ear alone.) The other group were treated with hormones.

Twenty-two of the women who had acupuncture treatment became pregnant, eleven after acupuncture, four spontaneously, and seven after appropriate medication. Twenty of the hormone group became pregnant, too, five spontaneously, and fifteen in response to medication.

It seemed that acupuncture was particularly helpful because it treated various disorders of the autonomic system as well, and the only side effects were seen with the hormone treatment. The authors considered that acupuncture offered a valuable alternative therapy for female infertility due to hormone disorders.

· *Adele* ·

I already had a son, conceived with no problems at all, when we wanted to have another baby. I became pregnant but had a miscarriage at eleven and a half weeks about which I was very upset, but because I had not felt quite right I thought that it was meant to be. I was not concerned about conceiving again because I thought I was good at getting pregnant, but it did not prove to be so easy. Eventually, after approximately three years of desperately trying to conceive, I did become pregnant again and because of the previous miscarriage had a very early scan at nine weeks. They could not find a heartbeat, and asked me to come back the following week. They still could not find one and concluded that it must have been a blighted ovum and said that I would have to come in for a D & C. I was desperately upset. I remember the nurses talking over my head saying, "What's she crying about?"

After I had had the termination I went back a couple of weeks later for a routine visit to the gynecologist. He explained that it had been a molar pregnancy, a hydatidiform mole, where cysts develop instead of a fetus and placenta. This distressed me considerably and I felt a great sense of anger for quite some time. The consequence was that I had to send a urine sample in a little bottle off by mail to the hospital at regular intervals for several months as hormone levels have to be followed up until they return to normal to make sure there is no risk of malignancy. I hated the impersonality of it, and my anger returned every time I had to send one of the urine samples. I was very relieved when they said that I could stop and start trying to become pregnant again.

However, it just didn't happen. I did have a couple of very early miscarriages when my period was two weeks late, but mainly I just did not conceive. I became very depressed and bitter. I found that there seemed to be pregnant women, a sight I found very difficult to cope with, everywhere I looked. I had various attempts at fertility treatment at conventional fertility clinics with no success, which served only to increase my depression.

A friend of mine suggested that I try acupuncture and recommended an acupuncturist who had treated her husband. I went to him and he treated me for infertility, eczema, and stress and also for hay fever but I still didn't get pregnant, although I kept on hoping. Then one day I suddenly got eczema really badly. I was visiting the acupuncturist every week or fortnight but the eczema did not improve. After a while my acupuncturist said he would treat me as the Chinese do and give me three treatments in a week for two weeks but charge me for only one until the eczema improved. In two weeks the eczema had gone.

By this time I had really given up. They say it only happens when you really give up, and I had bought myself a set of golf clubs and gone back to work, but all I ended up with was a job. We were really getting on, by now I was 46 and my husband was 60.

We went skiing and I felt sick, but I had done the year before and thought that it might have been something to do with the altitude. Then I found that although I was all right in the morning, I used to get incredibly tired in the afternoon. There was an old lady in my class who was raring to go and all I wanted to do was go to sleep. I did all sorts of things, like tobogganing, and then when I got back I started to wonder if I might be pregnant.

I went to a drug store other than the one I usually use and bought a pregnancy test. I hid in the bathroom from my cleaning lady and did the test, which proved positive! At that moment an accountant who was a friend of mine arrived at the house with a new client to talk over the client's case. The accountant was the first person I saw after I got the result. Much later he told me that the client had commented that I seemed to be a very cheerful girl.

I didn't tell anyone apart from my husband, the acupuncturist, and my gynecologist until I got the result of my CVS [chronic villus sampling—an early prenatal chromosome analysis] because I was so scared of the result. Then I told my son, who very much wanted a sibling. He said "Oh Mommy, I won't have to say "Je suis un enfant unique" in French class anymore."

It was a miracle. I just wasn't expecting it. Although my acupuncturist had never given up hope, I had. He said I was so strong there was no reason why I should not conceive, although I was not perhaps as fertile as I would have been at seventeen. The eczema treatment had not been specifically to improve fertility, but it worked. He nursed me through pregnancy and treated the baby through me at 14 and 26 weeks (moxabustion treatment is said to strengthen the baby, give it good digestion, and lots of hair), and has kept me going since.

The best thing about becoming pregnant was everyone else's reaction—they were all so pleased for us. The birth was no problem and now my younger son is nearly three and his older brother is fourteen. For us it was a real bonus that came when we were not expecting it.

· *Caroline* ·

I became pregnant with my first child almost embarrassingly quickly (at the first attempt, in fact) and I assumed it would be as easy the second time around. As I was in my mid-thirties, we thought we had better aim for a two-year gap and it was only after six months of trying that it began to dawn on us that there might be a problem. Luckily my GP was sympathetic and, in view of my age (by now all of 38!), referred me to a fertility clinic where I had an initial appointment within three weeks. However, after this encouraging start it was downhill all the way.

They ran all the usual tests on us, gave my husband the "all-clear," but discovered from blood tests that I was not ovulating, despite having regular periods. A course of Clomid was prescribed and this raised my hormone levels somewhat; but although one hospital doctor thought that "on balance" I was probably ovulating, I was convinced for several reasons that I was not. Six months after referral, impatient with seeing a different doctor each time—who often had not had time to read my notes beforehand—I postponed the laparoscopy they were urging on me and decided to try another approach.

A friend had had acupuncture, which she felt had helped her to conceive, so I made an appointment with the acupuncturist, whom I found very easy to talk to. After the consultation she told me, among other things, that my system was very sluggish and needed to be stimulated and balanced.

She asked me to go on a special diet for three weeks to sort out my digestive system. She also gave me needle treatment once a week and after the second treatment announced that I would be pregnant in three months. Being a natural sceptic (pessimist, my husband would insist), I really did not believe her: I suppose I did not want to let my hopes rise too much in case the treatment did not work after all. But she was right—three months later I was pregnant.

Acupuncture does hurt a bit, but only as the needles go in. Once they are in, you cannot normally feel them. And the slight discomfort of an acupuncture needle is nothing compared to the needles used for the countless blood tests demanded by the fertility clinic. The acupuncturist usually used between four and eight needles in a session. Most were in my feet, legs and hands, with occasional ones in my stomach—surprisingly, these didn't hurt at all.

I had a few treatments at specific times during my pregnancy to strengthen the baby. My acupuncturist also mentioned that if my baby became overdue, she could do an induction treatment to start the labor. I had hoped this would not be necessary, as my first labor started bang on time, but I was back at the clinic a week after my due date. A couple of hours after the treatment I felt that something was happening and fourteen hours later I was in labor. Katie was born after five and a half hours.

Perhaps the stress and depression caused by failing to conceive had had a negative effect, and simply doing something about it had made a difference. However, the same could have applied to the hospital treatment, which I had approached with high hopes, knowing several people who had conceived on Clomid. When we first started to try for our second child I was working, albeit part-time, in a job which was becoming increasingly stressful, and I am sure that giving up my job was a factor in our eventual success. Nevertheless, I am convinced that the acupuncture treatment was what finally did the trick.

· *Alison* ·

I had been married for eighteen months when I decided to stop the pill in order to become pregnant. When I stopped it, my periods stopped too, which had happened to me once before. As a result, I had a scan and was diagnosed as having polycystic ovaries. I was prescribed Clomid, which according to my gynecologist had no side effects, but when I looked at the instruction leaflet I was horrified. I took it to a pharmacist who seemed to know a bit more and after discussing it with him I decided not to take it.

At about this time my mother happened to meet the wife of an acupuncturist at her evening class and mentioned my problems to her. She suggested that I see her husband and so I made an appointment with him.

At the first appointment he told me that he felt there was a blockage within my system and said that he would treat it. After five or six treatments my periods started again—and then stopped. I was pregnant.

I went back to my GP, who was very interested. I've recommended acupuncture to a lot of my friends who just don't realize that there is an alternative to medical and surgical treatments for these sorts of problems. Several of them have endometriosis which has been treated by lasers, pills, and even hysterectomy, which is tragic if you want a baby. A friend of mine tried acupuncture for endometriosis and discovered that it really worked. She used to be in agony for ten days every month.

· *Aromatherapy* ·

Like nearly all alternative medical therapies, the use of essential oils and ointments to heal and improve well-being goes back to earliest time. Oils and ointments were used in rituals for religious purposes and therapeutically for treating illness, as well as in cooking. Vedic literature from India lists the use of more than 700 substances over 2,000 years before Christ, and the Chinese refer to aromatics in the details of their ancient herbal tradition recorded in *The Yellow Emperor's Book of Internal Medicine*, written at around the same time, a book which can still be bought today. An Egyptian papyrus dating from some 800 years earlier records the use of medicinal herbs and around 2000 B.C. the Egyptians were renowned for their use of oils and ointments, some of which, including cedar and myrrh, were used in the embalming process.

However, despite the widespread use of plants and spices in healing throughout many centuries, aromatherapy which is now well known and is growing in popularity, was only rediscovered in 1928 by a French chemist called Gattefosse. He was working in his family's perfume business and accidentally discovered the healing properties of the essential oil of lavender when he burnt his arm severely and plunged it into the oil, to find that it healed without scarring.

Essential oils of plants work in three different ways: pharmacologically, physiologically and psychologically. An essential oil can effect chemical changes within the body and reacts with hormones and enzymes. It also acts physiologically, by bringing about changes within the body—stimulating, sedating, and so on. Its physiological effect occurs when a person reacts to its smell.

Various combinations of oils are described as refreshing, uplifting, soothing, harmonizing, sensual, detoxifying, or good for aches and pains.

Not all plants yield essential oils, which are regarded as their life-blood and their defense against disease. Some release much more than others, which partly explains the difference in their prices; for example, it takes nearly half a ton of rose petals to make 100 grams of rose oil and 2 million jasmine flowers to make the same amount of jasmine oil. More information about the oils can be found in Chrissie Wildwood's *Encyclopedia of Aromatherapy* (see Further Reading).

Oils are prepared either by distillation or the application of pressure, which produces oils from such things as citrus fruits. Distillation is achieved by means of steam, water, or solvents.

Aromatherapy has been used successfully in the treatment of both male and female infertility. As with other alternative therapies, it is best to consult a qualified practitioner, who should be able to select the best combination of oils for your particular needs and provide an opportunity for relaxation as they are massaged into your body. Essential oils can also help with related problems, such as pelvic pain, painful and heavy periods, pain with endometriosis, and premenstrual syndrome.

An aromatherapist will take a full medical and emotional history and talk about why you have come. He or she will provide an opportunity to talk openly about your feelings and help you to cope if you fail to conceive. The aromatherapist can also provide aromatherapy to help with the stress of undergoing infertility treatment and supply oils for you to use at home, in the bath, or for massage, between treatments.

If you feel that you would like to try using essential oils, there are some that are recommended as being *especially* useful for fertility problems. When you buy essential oils for home use it is important to make sure that they are 100 percent pure oil, as some of those that are widely available are diluted (see pages 182 and 183 for suppliers).

There are various ways of using the essential oils, but apart from tea tree and lavender oils, they should be used in a carrier or base oil, otherwise they may irritate your skin.

How to use aromatherapy oils

Bath

Make a 6 percent blend by adding 6 drops of essential oil to a 5 ml teaspoon of base, which can be either whole milk or vodka.

This disperses the oil, which might otherwise sting or irritate. If your bath is acrylic or fiberglass you should wipe the oil off afterwards.

Massage oil

7–25 drops to 5 tsp base oil
3–5 drops to a 1 tsp base oil
20–60 drops to 7 tbsp base oil

Use oil such as sweet almond or grapeseed as a base and get your partner to massage it in. This will feel pleasant and ensure that the oils are absorbed into the bloodstream. You can also massage the oil into your skin yourself.

To aid fertility, one aromatherapist recommends a daily massage with the oils of your choice over the abdomen, hips, and lower back as far down as the crease in the buttocks. She says that women should start the treatment on the last day of their period, while a man can start at any time, but needs to persist for at least three months.

Compresses

Add a few drops of essential oil to a bowl of very hot or ice-cold water. Dip in a flannel or piece of cotton, squeeze it out, and apply to the affected area. Allow to cool or warm and repeat.

Vaporization

Add a few drops of oil in a bowl of warm water and place it on a radiator, or warm a little oil in a special burner or a metal ring, which can be placed over a light bulb. Alternatively, put a drop of oil on the corner of your pillow or on a handkerchief to smell during the day.

Infection

Pelvic and sexually transmitted diseases (for example, chlamydia) can be treated with essential oils, as they are powerfully antiseptic. Thyme, tea tree, pine, and eucalyptus oils are all recommended for the treatment of infection, and it is possible to have bacterial cultures tested to show which oils will kill the microbes involved. It would not be wise to treat these conditions without expert monitoring, but you may want to consider using them as an adjunct to antibiotic treatment or see an aromatherapist about treating the condition.

Aromatherapy oils

Experiment with the oils that appeal to you. Choose from the following to suit your particular problem.

Oils recommended for women:

rose—useful for regulating the reproductive system
geranium—regulates the menstrual cycle
bergamot—good for balancing the hormones
melissa—also regulates the cycle and is uplifting,
  so it is helpful when you feel depressed, as well

Also helpful for female infertility:

cypress	coriander
clary sage	geranium
thyme	fennel
nutmeg	Roman chamomile

Useful for both sexes, being relaxing, sedative, and aphrodisiac:

ylang ylang	bergamot
jasmine	rosemary
sandalwood	neroli

For male infertility:

thyme	sage
cumin	clary sage
basil	bergamot
cedarwood	black pepper
vetiver	geranium
angelica	

Experiment with mixtures that appeal to you.

· *Cranial osteopathy* ·

A cranial osteopath is a qualified osteopath who specializes in working on your whole body via the fluid and membranes of your brain and spinal cord. By working on the skull and pelvis, cranial osteopaths can assess the state of the connective tissue throughout the body and see where old traumas are preventing it from functioning properly. They are then able to remove the impediments which prevent those areas moving in time with the body's internal fluid tide. Correcting these will help you to function with a good flow of energy and a feeling of well-being and ensure that your body's involuntary mechanisms are working well.

The treatment involves lying on a couch for about 40 minutes while your head is held firmly. You may feel pressure and perhaps some subtle changes within it, but it is not painful. The osteopath may also put a hand under your pelvis to help assess your condition. You may feel light-headed for a few minutes after treatment.

A cranial osteopath is able to treat you structurally as well, correcting any malposition of your body by means of manipulation. Cranial treatment can be especially useful for treating women with fertility problems, as it can help the pituitary gland to function correctly. Those experiencing secondary infertility are particularly likely to benefit, because the cause of this problem may often be injuries sustained during the birth of the previous child. It is useful for relieving tensions held within the body too, and in so doing can allow fallopian tubes to regain their normal shape and any blockages to become unstuck. A few cranial osteopaths are also able to work directly on the pelvic area.

· *Allison* ·

I already had a daughter when I began to have problems conceiving, so I knew that I could have a child, but after eighteen months to two years of trying it wasn't happening.

I was referred to a gynecologist, who said that my progesterone levels were low and prescribed Clomid for me. I took it for three cycles and felt dreadful on it. I got migraines, which I had never had before, so badly that I was completely wiped out for three days of each cycle and had to hand over care of our daughter to my husband. At the time the drug was prescribed I asked the doctor if there were any side effects and he said there were very, very few and that the only one that I needed to know about was that it could result in my becoming pregnant with twins.

By the third cycle, when it still hadn't worked, I went to see a homeopath. She said that she would give me something to counteract the ill effects that Clomid was having on me and told me that it wasn't actually true that it had no side effects. She gave me something to read about it and how it could cause ovarian cancer and breast cancer. I was horrified and was on the verge of stopping it right then and there but thought that it would really screw things up if I stopped in the middle of a cycle. I wasn't prepared to take it any longer though.

I went back to the gynecologist who wanted to do more tests— laparoscopy, etc. He said it might be my husband's sperm count and gave me a bottle to produce a specimen for testing, but I thought that if it did prove low, my husband would feel guilty about it and it would be very unhelpful. At this point I decided not to have any further tests, if my progesterone level was low, so be it.

I tried to forget the whole thing, which is far easier said than done. I picked up a book which mentioned cranial osteopathy as a treatment for infertility. I had already taken my daughter to see Jill, a cranial osteopath, for being afraid of lying on her back and I thought it would be worth trying for me. I went along and Jill said that she found me quite tense, which I was aware of being, and she treated me but didn't find anything else specific. The homeopath had asked me whether I was stressed. I remember feeling very tired at times and wondering whether it was affecting me more than I realized. By the time I saw Jill I was really fed up and feeling low.

When I went back for an appointment a month later I was two weeks pregnant. I went twice more and she said that I felt very different. It was wonderful and too much of a coincidence for it not to be what helped, especially after two years of trying.

I know so many people with secondary infertility. You feel that you have a very low priority if you already have a child, even guilty about complaining, and that you shouldn't need any help. Many of those who do manage to conceive don't reach full-term.

The media portrays it as being so simple; you have a problem, you go to the doctor and it is miraculously fixed—except it isn't like that. I think that there is a lot more that we can do ourselves; it isn't only the gynecologist who can do something. We are not led to believe that we can empower ourselves. I'm so glad that I didn't have further investigations, but I'm probably more aware of the alternatives than most people I know. They just don't know they have a choice.

Allison's baby, Maria, was born quickly and happily at home, weighing 8 pounds 7 ounces.

· *Healing* ·

There have been healers as long as there have been people who need healing. Some people have the power to enable others to mend, purely by means of their touch or even by energy transference alone. There are many different terms for healing of this kind, including faith healing, spiritual healing, physical healing, therapeutic touch, and energy work. There is not necessarily a religious or spiritual link, although some healers do have spirit guides and may seem able to be in touch with the spirit world. You do not have to believe in healing for it to work: healers can help people who are not aware of their powers or are sceptical about them.

Treatment from a healer will involve discussing your problem and talking about yourself. Then the healer will ask you to sit in a chair or lie on a couch while he or she treats you. You may want to close your eyes, but keep them open if you feel more comfortable that way. The healer may put his or her hands on you (with your permission), or hold them above you, and move them over your body without touching you. The healer will receive an impression of the areas of your body which are not functioning well and use his or her energy to help them to improve.

As the healer treats your body you may feel warmth, heat, a tingling sensation, or a wave of energy in the part of your body which is being treated. You may not feel anything at all, but that does not mean that it is not working. Treatment may take half an hour or more, during which time you may feel relaxed, sleepy, or euphoric. When the treatment is over you may be feeling very relaxed and as if you are floating.

The effect of healing varies from person to person. If you are in pain at the time, you may find that the pain is lessened immediately. Sometimes your complaint may be exacerbated for a day or two and you may then become much better. You will probably feel better in between sessions, even if you have a condition which causes you physical pain.

Some healers charge nothing, some ask for donations and others provide healing on a professional basis.

· *Collette* ·

I have a baby girl of sixteen weeks after trying for seven and a half years. I probably tried almost everything, starting with visiting a person who was a reflexologist, an aromatherapist and a healer. She very quickly realized that I had a block in my spine around the area where the nerves feed the uterus. She said she was not surprised that I had not become pregnant but that I needed to see an osteopath to put my pelvis right before she could see me further.

She was right. When I was about 26 I had fallen down the stairs and cracked my coccyx and ever since then I had suffered from lower back pain. As all my family get backaches I didn't realize that my pelvis was so out—in fact, it took the osteopath to point out that one hip was higher than the other and that I was walking in a funny way. When I saw him he was able to put his finger on precisely the same spot that the reflexologist had identified. It was very painful when they touched it. The osteopath was able to straighten my back and the lower back pain improved enormously. I then went back to the first person I had seen.

In the meantime I tried acupuncture for a short time, mainly for catarrh, but it didn't help me get pregnant.

I did in fact become pregnant shortly after my spine was sorted out, but lost the baby at six to seven weeks. My healer realized that in fact the baby was not going to survive. It was very difficult for her—I was very excited about the pregnancy and she was trying to tell me that it wasn't properly attached and that she felt that things were not quite right.

However, she was a big help after the miscarriage as she was able to tell me that my grandparents were there beside me supporting me and that the tingle I felt was my grandmother stroking my hair. After that, although it was very emotional, the pain eased.

She was able to describe my grandparents perfectly; in fact, when I first went to see her, she told me my history without me saying anything. It was as if I had written it out and she was reading it. It let me know that she could really do it. It was really she who gave me the confidence to carry on and be sure that I would have a child. One time I was lying there in an altered state and I saw a child—almost as if it was in a film. It was in a garden and the child was laughing, really gurgling, right from the stomach and I remember wishing my husband could hear it because he really loves that noise that children make. As I came to, I was rather confused. The healer asked me what I had seen. I told her that I had seen a child, not thinking that it was my child, and she said, "that's your child, there is a child for you."

I knew she was right, because my mother had been to see her before I had and encouraged me to go. She told my mother that there were babies floating around her and said that there would be a baby in the family by Christmas. My mother was very excited on my behalf as she felt it would be mine as we had been trying so long. She knew that my sister's husband was about to have a vasectomy and my brother had a young baby so she thought it must be for me. In fact, my sister had become pregnant with her fourth child a week before the vasectomy was done.

No one ever found a medical diagnosis for my infertility; all our tests were fine, apart from my having a slightly raised prolactin level at one time. They treated me for that and then said that we were the same as everyone else. I found it harder that there seemed to be nothing apparently wrong—I cried when they told me the laparoscopy result was normal. Obviously, I was glad there was nothing really seriously wrong, but I had hoped there just might be a little something that they could put right.

We tried IUI for a year and then, in the middle of drug treatment, I developed a cyst. They stopped the treatment immediately, but we didn't want to waste the drugs and so tried and I conceived. The doctor didn't believe it was possible because I hadn't had the final injection to make the follicle rupture. Unfortunately, I miscarried and had three miscarriages altogether. It is easy not to realize how common they are, because people often don't talk about it, but if you say that you have had one, people will often say, "Well, actually it happened to me." Some people don't even realize that they are pregnant and may just consider it a nasty period that was a couple of weeks late, but with tests and being in tune with my body I've always been aware.

I'm sure that all the things I tried were helpful and have contributed to my feeling positive and relaxed, but the two things that helped most have been homeopathy and healing. I have a wonderful homeopath who is very easy to talk to and who helped me to prepare myself and balance myself until I felt I was ready for IVF. I could call him at any time and he was very helpful over the miscarriages.

I also have a friend who is an amazing healer who treated me. Every time I saw him it would give me a burst of energy, as if I had been plugged into an electric socket. He also helped me to talk about things; I talked to him a lot about dreams and other things that I didn't realize had affected me. He also does shiatsu and found that my heart center was agony when he touched it. He has taught my husband and me to be able to press each other's blocks and my heart center can now be pressed without causing pain. I'm now much more aware and can sense when I am developing blocks. The healer's powers are dramatic; you don't have to believe in him for it to work. He has convinced some very skeptical doctors that he can knit bones over a weekend. It takes a lot of energy but he can do it and they've actually proved it scientifically. Although they were incredulous, now quite a lot of them are lining up to be treated by him.

Eventually I felt strong enough and sufficiently balanced and positive to try IVF. I was supported by the homoeopath and healer and it worked the first time. I had progesterone to help ensure that I stayed pregnant and my homeopath gave me a wonderful herbal tincture to help prevent miscarriage. I took it regularly for the first four months and whenever I felt pains I would take some more *and they would go away. It helped with the morning sickness, too—I hardly felt sick; it was wonderful. The tincture was a very old remedy. He showed me the book it came from, which recommended it for women who were threatening to miscarry after falling out of a horse-drawn carriage. He said that there were no guarantees, but that he had never known anyone who had taken it to miscarry.*

I was helped by having the first four months off from work. I work as a nursery nurse with three- and four-year-olds and my manager kindly thought that I would stand a better chance of having a baby if I didn't work in the early months. I also started some more reflexology and was part-way through a course of self-hypnotism to help with the birth when I went into labor at 32 weeks. By then I had been doing yoga for three years and although it was a pity that I hadn't reached the end of the hypnotism course, because my husband missed his session and didn't know how to help me, I managed through a long labor which was of necessity drug-free because they didn't want any drugs to reach the baby. I was able to avoid a cesarean, which was on the cards at one point, and she was born a good weight for her gestational age: 4 lb 2 oz instead of the 3 lb to 3 lb 8 oz, which was expected. I knew that I would have her, but I just didn't know when and didn't expect it to take so long.

It is quite interesting to consider what delays pregnancy. I have a friend who was trying for five years. She was low in magnesium and corrected that, but it was when she overcame an emotional problem and forgave someone within the family that she became pregnant. She worked out for herself that that was what she needed to do and said it was like a weight had been lifted off her shoulders. She was pregnant within a week. Another friend desperately wants to be pregnant and has had all the tests, which showed nothing wrong. However, she lost her first baby from sudden infant death syndrome and when you really talk to her you realize that she is absolutely terrified of it happening again, and that it is easier for her not to be pregnant.

Luckily, my GP has been very supportive, although at one hospital the doctor thought even osteopathy was very cranky. I'd much rather try it that way than with drugs. My healer said that my aura while I was taking the IVF drugs was that of a person dying of cancer. He said he could see an inner core of strength and knew

*I was able to cope with it, and I felt better than I would have felt
without his energy, but he said that another healer would have just
noticed the damaging effect they were having. A friend I made
through IVF, whose attempt was not successful, is now trying out
things I did. People think she's crazy but it's worked for me. We
wish her and all the other couples still trying for a baby all the luck
in the world.*

· *Herbal medicine* ·

Herbs have been used for thousands of years. They are the old-
est form of medicine and they are still used to treat illness by
three-quarters of the world's population. The World Health
Organization (WHO) recognizes that for many people herbs
provide a safe alternative to imported Western drugs. They are
still used alongside mainstream drug treatment in Russia,
Germany, and China, where they are the primary source of help.
Herbal medicine, having been considered old-fashioned for
several decades, is now regaining popularity in the West, as people begin to appreciate its scope and range and realize that it
can be beneficial and far less harmful than taking prescribed
drugs.

Because herbs are used whole, instead of having their active
constituents extracted, they are far safer than drugs consisting
of plants from which the active ingredients have been isolated.
Each herb contains within it elements which will counteract the
potentially harmful effect of the active part of the plant. For
example dandelion, which acts as a diuretic, also contains potassium. Potassium is added to diuretic drugs to replace that which
is lost as a result of the drug's action on the body.

Treating infertility by means of herbs almost certainly
requires the help of a medical herbalist who is extensively trained
to treat people as a whole, considering all the emotional and cir-
cumstantial as well as physical problems that beset anyone in ill
health. An herbalist will take a full medical and personal history
and look at your lifestyle, diet, and environment. They will ask

about any vitamins, minerals or drugs that you might be taking, and make recommendations about any changes that might be necessary. They might then give you a combination of herbal tinctures to take several times a day and perhaps recommend that you delay trying to conceive for three months while your body is strengthened and made ready to enable you to conceive.

Although it is undoubtedly best to consult a medical herbalist directly regarding fertility problems, you may want to try some of the gentle herbs that are known to enhance fertility yourself. You might like to substitute herbal teas or infusions for ordinary tea and coffee, particularly if you are trying to reduce your caffeine intake. Herbs taken this way can complement any other therapy that you try and will help you to relax.

Herbs taken as teas as well as tinctures, encourage the circulation, improving drainage from the lymphatic system. They can restore regularity of the menstrual cycle and improve the tone and strength of the reproductive system. They may improve the male reproductive system too and will certainly benefit general health and well-being, but a man with a low sperm count might do best to consult a traditional Chinese herbalist (see page 139), as trials have shown that treatment with Chinese herbs can be of particular value in improving male fertility.

You can buy herbs ready prepared in liquid form as fluid extracts or tinctures as pills, or as powders which you can make into poultices or pastes or put into capsules yourself. Herbs are also made into creams and ointments. If you want to take herbs in these forms, consult a good book on herbs, such as *The Herbal Handbook* by David Hoffman (see Further Reading). If you want to take combinations of the herbs mentioned here, you can safely take them as infusions or decoctions which you can make with either dried or fresh herbs.

An infusion is made from the aerial parts of a plant, those parts which are above the ground, that is, the leaves, stalks, or flowers. It is made by putting either a teaspoonful of the dried herb or three teaspoonsful of the fresh herb in a container such as a teapot and then pouring on a cupful of boiling mineral water. This should be covered and allowed to stand for fifteen minutes without further heating. It can then be strained and drunk while still warm.

A decoction is made from the hard, woody parts of a plant—the roots, rhizomes, or stems. These need to be boiled in order to release their properties. Cut, chop, or crush the plant as much as possible before putting it into a stainless-steel or enamel saucepan. Add cold water, using 1 pint (660 ml) to 1 oz (25 g) of the dried herb, or 3 oz (75 g) of the fresh herb. Bring it to boil and then let it simmer for fifteen minutes or more. Allow it to infuse away from the heat and strain and drink it while it is still warm.

Both infusions and decoctions should be used within 24 hours, but they can be kept and reheated to a temperature below boiling.

Herbs for women

Herbs that are particularly useful for regularizing the female reproductive system are described below.

To balance hormones and correct an irregular cycle

Take the berries of the chaste tree, *Vitex agnus castus* (see Useful Addresses for sources of herbs). Pour a cup of boiling water on to 1 teaspoonful of the ripe berries and infuse them for ten to fifteen minutes. Drink the infusion three times a day, or take 1 to 2 ml of the tincture three times a day. This is also helpful with painful periods, PMS, and in the absence of periods. *Angelica sinensis* is recommended too.

For menorragia (excessively heavy periods)

Astringents are useful to treat this condition. They include American cranesbill, beth root, burr-marigold, lady's mantle, periwinkle, and shepherd's purse. You are also advised to include in your diet foods which are rich in iron, such as lean meat (especially kidney and liver), wheat germ, watercress, dried fruit, butter beans, kidney beans, dark-green vegetables, cream, cottage cheese, and unsweetened cocoa.

For painful periods

Black haw bark, cramp bark, and pasque flower are helpful.

For premenstrual tension

Scullcap combined with valerian, cramp bark, and pasque flower are valuable in treating premenstrual tension. Take dandelion to reduce fluid retention.

Pill-recovery herbs

Take one part each of black cohosh, chasteberry, liquorice and motherwort, and make up a tea, to be taken three times a day for the first two weeks, twice a day for the third week, and once a day for the fourth week. *Angelica sinensis* is also useful.

For infections of the reproductive system

The herbs that are required to treat infections include anti-microbials and alteratives (blood cleansers) to clear the lymphatic system, and astringents, which will help with mucus discharge.

Anti-microbials and alteratives include echinacea, garlic, wild indigo, cleavers, and poke root (poke root should not be used if there is any possibility you may be pregnant).

Astringents include American cranesbill, beth root, false unicorn root, life root, oak bark, and periwinkle.

These herbs can be made into an infusion or decoction and drunk three times a day. If you are not pregnant, the tea can also be used as a douche (douching is not recommended in pregnancy), and you may also be helped by taking 2 to 4 g of vitamin C daily and increasing your intake of garlic, ideally raw, but alternatively as garlic perles. Vaginal thrush can be improved by applications of live yogurt.

Herbs for men

Herbs which have a reputation for helping male fertility problems include damiana, ginseng and saw palmetto. They should be taken as infusions three times a day.

Stress and tension in both partners

Teas made from lime blossom, oats, or scullcap will help both partners and can be drunk freely.

· *Denise* ·

Allan and I decided to start trying for a baby in August 1992. I had been off the pill since we were married three years before and until then we had used barrier methods. However, five months before we planned to start trying I had a light period after 36 days followed by a heavy, painful, protracted one 19 days later. This was unusual as until then I had had normal periods regularly every 28 days. The period lasted so long that I went to my GP, who said that it was possible I could have had an early miscarriage. We were obviously quite shocked as we hadn't planned to start trying until the end of the summer, following a wedding at which I was to be bridesmaid and Allan was to be best man.

From then on my periods became very heavy and irregular. Quite concerned, I went back to my GP, who suggested I take a course of hormone tablets to try to regulate my periods. However, I wasn't eager to take them, so decided not to. In hindsight, I feel the tablets might have gotten my periods back to normal, but at the time I had no idea that I was going to have difficulty trying to conceive.

After the wedding, and after we had been trying to conceive, without success, for a couple of months, I went to my new GP (as we had moved to a new area) to discuss whether my awful periods could be having an effect on my fertility. He referred me to the local hospital but, due to a mix-up, I ended up in the subfertility unit rather than the gynecological unit as I had expected.

My first appointment with the consultant took place after we had been trying for five to six months. The consultant said that he normally started to investigate couples for infertility after they had been trying for a year, but since I was having menstrual problems, he would start investigating right away.

During the rest of 1993, the consultant carried out various routine tests on me—temperature charts, urine tests, blood tests to check hormone levels—all of which showed that I was ovulating. Allan was also tested and he proved to have a high sperm count with good motility. Although I was pleased that everything appeared to be normal, I was frustrated at not conceiving. During this time, I also started to consult a herbalist to try to help regulate my periods, with considerable success.

However, by February 1994 I was still not pregnant, so I was advised by the consultant to have a laparoscopy. It was at this point that I decided, for the time being, to go down the medical route alone, rather than contining to consult the herbalist as well, because I was anxious to find out whether the operation would reveal some physical irregularity that would need surgical correction. My herbalist respected my decision and asked me to keep her informed of the outcome.

The laparoscopy showed that one tube was slightly blocked but not so badly that it would prevent an egg passing through; the other tube was fine. I left the hospital feeling quite optimistic. I was given Clomid to take for the next three months. However, I was only able to take it for one month as I developed horrible side effects with disturbed vision. It felt as if my eyesight was shutting down and I became completely disoriented. I was advised by the consultant to stop taking Clomid immediately.

In May of the same year I had an hysterosalpingogram [HSG], which showed that everything was fine. There appeared to be no evidence of a blockage, as the dye was flowing through perfectly. It was rather a humiliating experience lying exposed from the waist down on the table, while a nurse held on to my arms so that I would not jerk when the doctor inserted the dye through my cervix. However, I felt more embarrassed by the presence of the elderly male radiographer, who was dressed as though he were a country gentleman. After the radiographer had finished his part in the procedure, he left the room, leaving the door open to a busy corridor. I was furious, as I had not been covered up. My anger was compounded by the fact that Allan was not allowed in to accompany me.

After the HSG, we were put on the waiting list for IUI [Interauterine Insemination], which I understood would take about a year. However, Allan and I were reasonably optimistic that I would become pregnant naturally. The next year was dreadful. Every month I had a period, which I found so distressing. I couldn't understand why, if Allan and I were perfectly healthy, I was unable to conceive. I felt like a failure.

Then, in February 1995, I went to see a reflexologist. Apart from the wonderfully relaxing reflexology sessions, the reflexologist advised Allan and me to eat as much organic food as we could find, which we did. We had a bag of organic vegetables delivered every two weeks and we also managed to find a lot of other organic food at the local supermarket, flour, cereals, yogurt, milk, etc. We discussed diet at length and the possibility that I might be getting too many estrogens from non-organic food. My reflexologist also gave me some Australian bush and Bach flower remedies to help me emotionally and recommended I take some vitamins and minerals. After a few sessions, coincidence or not, I became pregnant.

Unfortunately, I miscarried at six weeks. Allan and I were devastated. It just didn't seem fair—I felt as if we had been robbed. I did go to a bereavement group for parents who had lost babies but everyone there had conceived without difficulty, although they may have had recurrent miscarriages. I felt I didn't really fit in. Although one part of me was relieved that I could become pregnant, after doubting it could happen for so long, there was also nagging doubts: maybe that had been my one chance to become pregnant; perhaps it would take me as long again to become pregnant and I might then miscarry in any case. I was in a dreadful state. Although Allan and I were still on the waiting list for IUI, we saw this as a last resort.

From that point on, with every period I became more and more depressed, especially as most of my friends subsequently became pregnant. It seemed that each month, as soon as I had come to terms with the onset of my period, another one of my friends or family announced they were pregnant. They found it hard to tell me as they knew how upset I would be. Every month I would get my hopes up, being careful with what I ate and drank, not taking pain killers for headaches, etc. in case I was pregnant, and every month I was bitterly disappointed.

Finally, in October, seven months after the miscarriage, there came a turning point. Allan and I were due to go to dinner with friends we hadn't seen for awhile. My period was late, so before we went out I did a pregnancy test. It was negative and I was very upset. We summoned the energy to go out. We had only been at our friends' house a short while when my friend announced that she was five and a half months pregnant—believe it or not, I hadn't noticed her bump! I could feel myself go hot and a lump appeared in my throat. Thank goodness I was able to hide my distress behind my wineglass. I somehow managed to say all the right things, although I don't know how I got through the evening. That weekend I had a mini breakdown. I cried and cried—I was inconsolable. I couldn't understand why it wasn't happening for us, why I did not seem to be functioning properly, how my friends were able to get pregnant without difficulty. I felt I was not a complete woman. Allan was marvelous and was a great support.

However, this did seem to be a turning point, as from then on I decided to take charge of my life and shift its focus. I had put my life on hold. I was in a job I hated, but I felt I had been biding my time until I became pregnant. I had to try to accept that we might not have a baby. I had recently passed an A-level in English Literature, which had boosted my morale, so I decided to apply to a local university to do a full-time history degree, for which I was accepted. I also went back to the herbalist. She encouraged me to continue eating organic and free-range foods and also put me on a course of herbs. She recommended that I didn't try to become pregnant for three months to give the herbs a chance to work. This was very hard. I continued to also take multivitamins and folic acid and carried on with the reflexology sessions twice a month.

The three months were up in December 1995. We tried again and I conceived right way. It was an anxious time—I was very concerned that I would miscarry again—but , finally, I gave birth to my beautiful son, Matthew, in October 1996.

I really believe that natural therapies helped me to become pregnant. Reflexology helped me to relax, which is half the problem. I couldn't relax because I was so stressed every month. Coincidentally, the consultant had informed us on our last visit to the hospital that they were considering employing a homeopathic doctor because they recognized what a big part stress had to play in the cause of infertility. In my case, I feel he was definitely right.

· *Emma* ·

We first started trying to have a baby in 1990. When it didn't happen I had all the usual tests and then, although they were not conclusive, I found that I was being channeled down the IVF route with disconcerting rapidity.

At the first hospital that we attended I was given a laparoscopy *and was told that one tube was blocked and that this meant both would be blocked—it was bilateral. I couldn't understand why and then was given a hysterosalpingogram. When it was performed, the operator said, "Which tube is meant to be blocked? Dye is spilling from both of them." When I told the doctor this, he said "It doesn't mean anything at your age." We were also told that my husband had sperm antibodies. We asked how this would affect his chances of parenthood and were told that they didn't really know.*

As a result we were referred to another teaching hospital as they said IVF was our only hope, and I had another laparoscopy. This time they said one tube was caught up but the other one was all right. Because of this, they described us as suffering from unexplained infertility. We asked about the antibodies again and I was more or less told not to worry my pretty little head about it. I found the whole experience agonizingly frustrating; I really felt that they were treating a body, not a person. I remember once asking to be involved with the treatment and they were astonished that I should have spoken.

We did ask if there was anything that we could do to help ourselves, by way of diet or lifestyle changes that we should make, and they said no. I was concerned that my husband's smoking and drinking could be adversely affecting his chances, but they wouldn't commit themselves, whereas he really needed a doctor to tell him to stop.

I was given a treatment to prepare me for IVF. This was done for three consecutive cycles, although it is apparently good practice to allow three months between each attempt. The first two had to be abandoned because I did not produce any follicles and the third time they did get as far as egg collection, only to discover that although there were 2–3 follicles they contained no eggs. I was on very high doses of Pergonal—eight to ten capsules a day—and all for no result. The Pergonal was to stop hot flashes, though, and I felt that I was able to monitor how well they were regulating my body by its response and told them that I could tell if I needed more. They said that they weren't able to go on my feelings about my body and when the third attempt failed, they just recommended a fourth attempt. I said that I would like to go away and think about it, as I had a job and so on.

Fortunately I had met a girl at one of those awful evenings that they held so that would-be-parents could listen to eminent doctors and occasionally get the chance to talk to each other. She said that she knew of a wonderful herbalist/midwife and gave me her details. By the time the end of the cycle of the third attempt came I was still getting hot flashes and I was afraid that they had put me into menopause. They say that it is not possible, but I know plenty of people to whom it has happened.

So I made an appointment and went to see the herbalist. I had started the IVF in January and finished in August and went to see her in September, when I was almost 42. She said that the first thing to do was to stop the hot flashes, which she managed to do with her sage teas within seven days. They stopped quite suddenly. Then she said that I needed to cleanse my system of all these drugs and made me eat nuts and liquorice and take teas and potions, all of which I did. Best of all, she encouraged me: she said it wasn't hopeless and that other women in their forties had children.

She was always encouraging and really managed to get through to my husband. She said that she needed to treat us both but he was very resistant to the idea. He felt threatened and inadequate because it was so sensitive. He was completely detached about the business; he could cope if I had to have treatment but got very angry if he did. He resisted going to see the herbalist for ages and kept missing or breaking appointments. Finally I managed to get him there one Saturday morning and he almost refused to go in. I thought that he would be out again within a couple of minutes and I waited for him in the car. Minute after minute ticked by and he eventually emerged after one and a half hours. I don't know what she said to him, but she not only managed to persuade him to stop drinking and give up smoking but he also changed his diet and became much more conscious of what he ate. He was also persuaded to take the horrible-tasting herbal medicines that she prescribed.

We changed clinics again, having found the hospital an awful experience. The next doctor was much more helpful and prescribed steroids for my husband, which the last hospital had refused to give him. By the second month I was pregnant.

A lot of things came together at the same time. Our herbalist was so helpful and we are incredibly grateful for what she did for us both as a couple. The whole experience was so soothing, at a time when things were getting very tricky. It was stressful having

*to have sex by the clock and she was able to tell me that it was nor-
mal for men to get headaches because they knew it meant so much
to you. I was able to see her during my pregnancy and then she
attended to me in labor. She came to our home and then went with
us to the hospital. She gave me things to take in labor—herbal
medicines and funny little drinks. I had a fantastic labor and eventually had Rachel by ventouse. I was the only one of my prenatal
group of fifteen who was able to sit down after giving birth and I
am sure that was due to the herbs I was given.*

*I was pleased to encounter the consultant who had told me that
I would never have a baby except by IVF one day when I had my
daughter with me. I was able to tell him that she had been conceived naturally. "Best way," he said.*

· *Chinese herbal medicine* ·

The use of herbs in Chinese medical treatment is, like other
herbal medicines, centuries old. It differs from Western herbal
medicine in the nature of the herbs involved, which may be
grown only in China, and the fact that it is often used in conjunction with acupuncture. In addition, the Chinese regard the
boundaries between herbal medicine and food as being less
distinct, so specific foods may be recommended as part of the
treatment, oysters or lamb's kidneys, for example. A particular form of older Chinese herbal medicine was known as "Eat
medicine." Even today, the Chinese will prepare various foods
as a medicinal remedy for the whole family and it is believed
that some foods should be eaten only at certain times of the
year. This is regarded as preventative medicine, and is not the
same as having medicinal herbs in soup form to treat specific
ailments.

In China, herbs may be taken in combination—up to twelve
per combination—and they may be prepared as soups or teas
or supplied in preparations which are available for purchase
as pills, ointments, or liquid medicines. There is a greater
recognition of the value of herbs in everyday life. To treat a
headache, for example, the Chinese person tends to buy an herbal

remedy, either as ready mixed dried herbs or in pill form, just as a Westerner might buy a bottle of Tylenol.

If you consult a Chinese herbalist, you will find that he or she will first examine you in a similar way to an acupuncturist (many will be qualified to treat you in both ways). The routine examination involves four things: asking, looking, listening, and feeling. Asking means taking a full medical history and finding out about your lifestyle, diet, sex life, fears, and upbringing. Looking involves observing the color of your face, your general body type, your way of speaking, the appearance of your tongue (regarded as an internal organ and very important in diagnosis), your apparent mental state, and your facial expression. The herbalist will listen to your breathing, coughing, voice, and smell (smell is part of the listening examination) and finally feel your pulses, as in acupuncture.

When the herbalist has decided where your deficiencies or excesses lie, he or she will prescribe herbs to restore the balance within you. These may be dried herbs which you have to make into a soup at home following instructions carefully, or you may be prescribed a patent remedy. You may be given a repeat prescription, or be asked to come back after a week or so. You may also be advised not to drink tea, which is regarded as an herb in its own right. The herbal prescription will vary according to your size, age, normal health, whether herbs or minerals are being prescribed, where you live and work, and whether or not the necessary herbs are strong-tasting. Boiled herbs are prescribed in much larger quantities than those in pill, powder, or tablet form. You may also be treated with moxabustion (see page 112), or be recommended to take up Qi Gong—a form of Chinese exercise or try meditation, massage, or biofeedback.

Some examples of female prescriptions are: Tang Kuei and Paeonia Formula, White Phoenix Pills, Women's Precious Pills, Lycium Formula and Cinnamon and Hoelen Formula. Treatment for men could include Ginseng-Astragalus Sperm-supporting tablets, Lower Stamen Combination, Ginseng and Ginger Combination, Right Restoration Pills, and Five Seed Numerous Offspring Pills.

There is more research evidence available regarding Chinese (and Japanese) herbal medicine than there is for Western medical herbalism, and the results, particularly for male infertility, look impressive. One study[2] treated eight couples who had anti-sperm and/or antizonal pellucida antibodies in their blood serum (diagnosed as Kidney Yin Deficiency—Hyperactivity of Fire Syndrome) and treated them with Zibai Dihuang Pills, a recipe of Chinese medical herbs. The treatment made the antibodies negative in 81 to 83 percent of the couples and pregnancy followed in all of them between one and nine months after treatment. Another study[3] described using composite Wuzi Dihuang liquor to treat male infertility. It is indicated in mild and medium oligozoospermia. The treatment was effective in 84 percent of cases, but not when the patients had severe oligospermia, azoospermia, a testicular volume of 15 ml or less, or endocrinologic or chromatic abnormality. Experimental studies showed it significantly increased the percentage of reproductivity in mice and could directly safeguard the sperm of male infertility patients.

A particularly impressive-sounding study, which unfortunately gives insufficient detail,[4] describes how 202 cases of male infertility were treated with Shengjing pill. After treatment, quantity and quality of sperm were significantly improved, levels of FSH, LH, and testosterone were enhanced to normal in 96 patients, and levels of anti-sperm antibody were reduced to normal in 45 out of 148 cases followed up. Of the partners, 116 became pregnant and have had 108 well-developed babies.

Another trial, which employed Japanese herbal medicine,[5] suggested that Hochuekkito corrected Leydig cell dysfunctions in some men, resulting in improvements in sperm quality.

Women with endometriosis were treated with Nei-Yi recipe in one study. It was found to increase plasma beta-endorphin levels, which were lower in women with moderately and severely painful periods, (particularly in the luteal phase and in those with pelvic pain) than in control subjects and women with mild pain. Nei-Yi recipe raised levels significantly.[6]

· *Catherine* ·

I had been trying to become pregnant for about fifteen months when I visited a Chinese herbalist. Tests that I had done three months before showed that I was ovulating properly and I was just about to persuade my husband to have his sperm assessed when I went to the herbalist in order to get help with giving up smoking. I didn't even mention the problems we were having in conceiving, but he felt my pulse and announced that I was a very stressed-out person. I hadn't thought that I was, but he gave me ten pills to take in the morning and another ten at night, and I certainly started to feel very relaxed. I managed to stop smoking for awhile and it was probably the most effective therapy that I have tried.

We then went on vacation. I didn't want to become pregnant then because I wanted to be able to have a drink and enjoy myself. However, to my complete surprise, especially as it was at a time when I should not have been ovulating, I found that I was pregnant. After a healthy pregnancy, I had a little boy, who was conceived within a month of starting the treatment.

· *Homeopathy* ·

Homeopathy, like most complementary therapies, is a method of helping the body to heal itself. It was introduced in 1796 by a German, Samuel Hahnemann. By chance, he discovered that when he gave minute doses of drugs which mimicked the symptoms of an illness to people who actually had the disease, they recovered. For example, consuming cinchona bark will, for a short while, give you the symptoms of malaria, but, taken in a very dilute preparation, it will cure the disease. This is known as "Let like be cured by like," which is the philosophy on which homeopathy is based.

Hahnemann tried out large numbers of substances on his family and friends and, by noting their reactions, was able to build up a large repertory of treatments or remedies. In homeopathic terms, symptoms of illness are seen as the body's reaction to illness and its attempts to overcome it. Homeopathic remedies strengthen that reaction so that the body can overcome the disease and heal itself.

Homeopathic treatment is specially tailored to each individual. If you consult a homeopath, he or she will pay particular attention to the sort of person you are: your constitution, coloring, likes and dislikes, what makes you feel better or worse, what sort of temperament you have and what your energy levels are like. When they have a good picture of you—and the initial interview may last for as long as an hour and a half, they will think hard about the right remedy to treat you. Because the treatment is chosen expressly for you, you may get a different remedy from someone with identical problems. For this reason, it is necessary to consult a homeopath in person. When they know you personally, it may be possible to consult them about your problems by telephone.

The remedies, unlike pharmaceuticals, are extremely dilute and, paradoxically the more dilute they are, the more powerful they are said to be. Most are derived from plant material, although some are prepared from things like gold and sand which are generally regarded as inert. They are prepared by serial dilution from a mother tincture which is made from the herb mashed in water. One drop of the tincture is diluted with 9 or 99 drops of the diluting medium, depending on whether the potency is to be decimal (x) or centesimal (c). The mixture is shaken vigorously and then one drop from that mixture is taken and diluted again in the same ratio. The first dilution becomes 1c or x, the second 2c or x and so on. The potency that is most widely available in shops is 6c, although the c may be missing from the name on the label, so that it appears as Arnica 6, for example. The names are often abbreviated too, Antimonium tartrate may be known as Ant tart, for example.

The fact that the original substance has been so diluted means that it is quite safe to take remedies based on things which in their undiluted form are poisonous, such as arsenic. The remedies are also particularly good for treating children and for use in pregnancy when conventional medicines are best avoided.

Homeopathy and infertility

Both partners should be treated as it is considered important that you should both be in optimum health preconceptually. There are remedies to treat both male and female infertility, depending on the cause of the problem. For instance, folliculinum might be prescribed for a woman whose menstrual cycle has been disordered by taking the pill, or sepia or pulsatilla to strengthen her reproductive system. Some remedies are designed to target the uterus or ovaries. Either sex may be found to have a chemical imbalance for which homeopathic preparations of tin, iron, or calcium might be prescribed. You might be given a homeopathic remedy made from an unusual chemical that was adversely affecting you.

On a mental and emotional level, the homeopath will try to discover whether any blocks are holding you back and treat them if necessary. They can also treat you in an effort to prevent your prospective children from inheriting family tendencies towards heart disease, TB, cancer, etc. A homeopath will also look at your lifestyle and make recommendations about not burning the candle at both ends, for instance, and examine smoking and drinking habits.

Some homeopaths will work with people while they are taking fertility drugs, while others will not. They feel that the prescription fertility drugs can be too strong and heavy for homeopathic remedies to work against; if taken every month they may negate the effects of the homeopathic treatment.

The remedies

The remedies themselves come in different strengths. The lower dilutions, such as 6c or 30c, are generally used for physical problems, while the higher, more powerful ones tend to be used for emotional problems. It is felt that it is more important for the remedy to be right than to be concerned about the potency. You may be given a single tablet only, or several to take in a day. When acute conditions are being treated at home, you can take tablets frequently until the condition improves, but for long standing and serious conditions they need to be prescribed for you.

As with reflexology, the condition may briefly get worse before it gets better. This is known as aggravation and may manifest as a skin rash, or you may develop a whole series of symptoms, including those you have had before, so that it is like a film of your ill health running backwards. After this there should be a big improvement as your body starts to mend.

The tablets come as hard or soft tablets or powders which should be allowed to dissolve under the tongue. They should be taken in a clean mouth, which means that you should not have anything to eat or drink for about 20 minutes before or after taking the remedy. You should avoid coffee and peppermint while you are using homeopathic remedies. You may need to buy a special toothpaste especially for homeopathy users. It is also thought inadvisable to use an anti-perspirant, although a simple deodorant is fine. You should avoid essential oils of black pepper, camphor, eucalyptus or any of the mints, because they can antidote the remedies too.

The medicines are sensitive and can easily become contaminated, so they should be stored in a cool dark place well away from strong smells. Keep them in their original containers and tip the pills out into the lid when you want to take one so that you don't touch any that need to be put back. The remedies can also be taken in warm water; this is particularly suitable for acute conditions where doses need to be taken frequently. Crush two tablets and dissolve them in warm water and sip it slowly.

To find a homeopath, contact the National Center for Homeopathy or Homeopathic Educational Services (see page 180) or talk directly to a homeopathic college.

Two studies on the effect that homeopathy can have on treating infertility were published in Germany in 1993. One took 21 women with infertility caused by hormonal disorders and matched them with another group of women with the same problems so that they were of similar age, period of infertility, weight, type of disorder, etc. and treated one group with homeopathy and the other group with hormones. Six pregnancies occurred in each group, but all six of the homeopathic group went on to have a baby, while four of the hormone group miscarried. Homeopathy seemed superior as a form of treatment because it eliminated the hormone disorders in 50 percent of the group and in 19 percent various functional disorders improved. Transient side effects were noted in 10 percent of the women. In the drug-treatment group, their general condition was not improved and it even deteriorated in 29 percent of them. Homeopathic treatment was ten times cheaper than the drug treatment.[7]

The other study[8] examined 119 women with infertility due to hormonal disorders. They were all treated with homeopathy and 25 became pregnant; all but two pregnancies went to full-term.

· *Jo* ·

We started trying for a baby almost as soon as we got married. We stopped using contraception and assumed that we would become pregnant, as everyone else was. After we had been trying for about a year we started to get a bit concerned. I was 31 by then and, although that is not very old, we knew that if you had difficulties it was better to get them sorted out sooner rather than later.

Then I had an awful accident falling down an escalator. I damaged my arm very badly and had to have four operations and was in the hospital for two weeks. It took quite a long time to get over it and I was off work for a long while, so although we were still not using contraception we had other things to think about.

By this time I was seeing a nutritional specialist to make sure that I was eating well so that I would be fit enough to become pregnant. Around this time Philip had a sperm count. He has always looked after himself very well, but it came back as being very low: 50 percent of the sperm were abnormal and we were told they were unable to account for 30 percent, which left only 20 percent of not very many. Philip asked the doctor what he could do and was told to wear boxer shorts, not to smoke or drink and get some exercise. As this was the way he lived anyway, it was not much help.

By then I was also seeing a homoeopath, mainly to deal with the aftereffects of the accident, but she also started treating both of us individually for our problems in becoming pregnant. I had had a long history of PID in my twenties and one way or another it began to look as if we had no hope of pregnancy without a great deal of medical intervention, but she kept giving us different remedies that she said would help. She told Philip not to get caught up on the question of numbers but to concentrate on the quality, and gave him things to help him loosen up medically and physically. She would say: "And this is helpful for getting you ready for pregnancy."

Our doctor referred us to a hospital fertiltiy clinic but there was a waiting-list of seven months for fertility treatment. We were still being treated by the homeopath and went to the clinic really wondering if we were certain that we wanted to go through with it. I realized that it takes over your whole life and I wondered whether we really wanted to do that and whether it would work. We had been under a lot of stress; my mother had just died and I questioned whether we should be doing it.

The first appointment was with a lovely consultant. We went straight in to see him and he explained that there would be six months of tests and then possibly another six months while they decided what to do and so it might be a year before we had any treatment. We had to book the tests ahead to make sure that they coincided with my periods. We used to have sex all the time; now it had to be regulated to fit in with all the tests. Then I was admitted for the test where they inject blue dye into your fallopian tubes. I had to take antibiotics for a week before that and then for a week afterwards. They said that it wouldn't hurt, but they also gave me a sheet explaining that the test could be quite uncomfortable and that you would need someone to be with you and drive you home, so I knew it would be agony. In fact, I didn't have the test in the end. I did go along to have the internal scan done (by what seemed to be an eighteen-year-old) and to have my blood tested.

I went along with a smile on my face hoping to talk to other people about their experiences, and came across a huge waiting-room full of people looking dead miserable. There was no eye-contact; I couldn't talk to anyone. They all had bowls full of vials of hormones or blood samples. I don't think that I am exaggerating; there was a *real feeling of despair, and I feared that I could see myself like that in three months time.*

It was very traumatic and we only scratched the surface of it. You're not told very much. We were working out whether we could manage to do the injections ourselves and, if not, how I could get to the hospital to have them done by the practice nurse, when our GP asked who was going to pay for it. It had never occurred to us to think about who would pay for the drugs and the treatment and we had to go and see the woman at the hospital who deals with those things. No one had told us about it, or that we stood a better chance if we put in our bid at the start of the financial year, before the budget had been allocated.

I had the preliminary tests and was about to have the hysterosalpingogram when I started to feel very peculiar and my period was late. I was normally extremely regular, even to the day. I did two pregnancy tests, one on the Tuesday and one on the following Friday, and they were both negative. I started to get distressed because I needed my period to start before I could start taking the antibiotic prior to the blue-dye test.

Then I went to a party for my father's seventieth birthday and the next day wanted to talk to my relatives—I do enjoy talking— but felt I just couldn't be bothered. I told my cousin, who suggested that I do another pregnancy test and it was positive.

I phoned the clinic and they said "Come in" and were lovely. I think they can count me as a success in their statistics, even though I hadn't started treatment.

I'm convinced that it was the homeopathy that did it. I went on seeing the homeopath all through pregnancy and she was able to treat me for all those unpleasant ailments like heartburn and hemorrhoids completely successfully. I took remedies in labor until I had the cesarean and Mia, five weeks old yesterday.

· *Eleanor* ·

I had a daughter, conceived naturally, and when she was about four I thought it would be great to have another one. I had a miscarriage and then after that I failed to become pregnant despite using no contraception. After three years of trying, I mentioned it to one of the doctors I was seeing and she gave me Clomid. It made me feel pretty bad—I get PMT anyway and it made me feel as though I had it all the time. I felt completely awful for about three months. It was while I was taking it that I saw a program about Clomid which mentioned the fact that the chance of having a multiple birth as a result of taking it was 8 or 9 percent. I was horrified, as I didn't want twins or more, or to be faced with selective abortion.

After about a year I finally got an appointment at a fertility clinic. There I was prescribed more Clomid and I thought, to heck with it, I'm not going down that path, so I asked my doctor to refer me to a homeopath. He referred me to someone at another hospital who was a GP who had retrained as a homeopath. I first went to see her one and a half years ago. By that time we had been trying for a baby for four years. She gave me a couple of constitutional remedies but said she would make no promises.

I had always had irregular periods, perhaps having one every other month. This seemed to be completely irrelevant to the doctors at the infertility clinic. I could have been talking about my toenails for all the interest they took—all they wanted to do was bombard my womb with Clomid, dishing them out like Smarties. It was very unspecific to myself.

As I took the remedies I started to feel things happening. I had a period nearly every month and found that I was also undergoing mental changes. I could feel some order coming into my life. Other things were not so comfortable. I had a big breakout on my skin, for example. I went to see the homeopath two or three times and then I got pregnant. It took me ages to realize—I thought I had prolonged PMS, as I could miss periods for weeks normally, although I had felt things happening in my cycle. I saw her twice during my pregnancy, which was great as well. I had a drug-free labor and gave birth to a lovely baby boy two months ago, nine years to the week since I had my first child. They say that you have to give up hope and then it happens—you just relax. Just before I conceived I really did think, Maybe it will never happen.

Magnus is an exceptionally happy and healthy baby and I'm sure this is considerably due to the way I was able to look after myself during pregnancy and in the early days after birth.

I think you have to trust your instinct and choose the things that you feel are right for you. It's terribly unscientific, but I think *you know what works for you; we've been taught to mistrust our intuition, but you have to use intuition all the time when you have a child.*

· *Hypnotherapy* ·

Hypnotherapy is able to treat infertility, particularly in women, although it may be useful for men too. It may seem hard to believe that the subconscious mind can actually have an effect on the fallopian tubes so that it prevents them working to propel the egg downwards, but hypnotherapists have proven success in treating unexplained infertility. This is because they are able to reach a person's subconscious and access the mental or emotional blocks which may be preventing conception. It has been shown that women who, for whatever reason, have formed very unfavorable ideas of pregnancy and childbirth, can erase these ideas and have them replaced with positive, favorable impressions while under hypnosis. Some hypnotherapists believe that spasmodically blocked tubes (those that are not physically blocked but are subject to spasm) relax after hypnotherapy, when the woman's fears and anxieties have been treated and her self-esteem enhanced.

Hypnosis works in several ways, but it can only work with your consent. You are neither asleep nor unconscious while you are being hypnotized and the hypnotherapist cannot control your mind or behavior against your will. You can be hypnotised only if you agree to it and want it to work. A hypnotherapist will help you reach a state of deep relaxation and enable you to concentrate intensely on a limited area of attention. You will find that you have a heightened level of responsiveness to suggestions, cues, or signals made by the therapist. Your critical faculty will be reduced, so that it seems as though you have no previous experience of the subject and thus will be able to take suggestions at their face value.

In treating female infertility, a hypnotherapist will discuss your history and the difficulties you have experienced and then perhaps inquire about your relationship with your partner. They may then induce hypnosis merely by talking soothingly to you, possibly talking about the reproductive system and the process of fertilization and reminding you that there are no physical impediments to your becoming pregnant. The therapist may describe the way in which the egg is propelled down the fallopian tubes by tiny muscular movements or pulsations of the small muscles which surround the tube. You may be asked to visualize this and then to appreciate that the tightening of your muscles was narrowing the tubes so that the egg could not be propelled along it. The hypnotherapist may then ask you visualize these muscles gradually relaxing to the point where the fallopian tube is sufficiently wide to allow the egg to move down it, and encourage you to count downwards to yourself as the muscle around the tube relaxes until it is fully open.

During the session the therapist will also provide supporting and comforting images of becoming pregnant and the process of childbirth. They will endorse the belief that you will become pregnant, and also find out if anything in your past might be blocking pregnancy. If that is the case, they will be able to eliminate the fear or anxiety by rationalizing it and replacing it with positive images. You will be given instructions and perhaps a tape-recording of your session so that you can repeat the process several times a day while you are at home.

Additional benefits of hypnotherapy are that it can improve your morale and self-confidence and make you feel more optimistic; and it has no side effects.[9]

A description of the successful treatment of four women, two of whom had secondary infertility, is contained in one study. The periods of infertility had lasted for six years for one woman, four years in two, and two years for the last. Each woman had six sessions of hypnotherapy treatment spaced over different intervals of time. The woman with two years infertility attended a crash course for a week, as she lived elsewhere, and was pregnant six months after the last session. Another was found to be pregnant after five weeks of treatment, having tried to conceive for four years. The next woman, who had also been infertile for four years, became pregnant during the course of her treatment but, sadly, miscarried at ten weeks, while the last became pregnant five weeks after the final session of her course of treatment, which lasted three weeks. Interestingly, the second woman had attended for help to stop her biting her nails, not being aware that hypnotherapy might be able to help her infertility. She had a normal delivery of a healthy boy—and stopped biting her nails.[10]

Also of interest is an older work discussing treatment of infertility in women who had pain on intercourse. In most cases the period of infertility was shorter, but all eight women conceived within fourteen months, several quite quickly.[11]

· *Sophie* ·

We started trying for a baby in 1991, when we got married. After the first four months, it seemed as nothing was happening, so I went to the doctor and it turned out that I was not ovulating. He said I should be put on Clomid, but as my pap smear showed abnormal cells, he said we should wait. Three months later the smear was still abnormal and a very mild cervical dysplasia was diagnosed, but nothing was to be done and I was still not allowed to take Clomid.

In January 1992 I went into the hospital to have a laser vaporization to treat the dysplasia as all doctors seemed to want to get it out of the way before I got pregnant. Three months later my pap smear still showed abnormal cells, but this time the doctor said I could take Clomid. After five months of taking it (with no side effects, I must say), I became pregnant. Unfortunately, the pregnancy was ectopic. I had already had a scan at about six weeks and the doctor said that he could not see anything in the uterus but that it might be too early to see it. He didn't warn me to be aware of any abdominal pain because of the risk that it could be ectopic. As it was my first pregnancy, I was not aware of the significance of the pain I started to feel, so I put up with it until the third day, by which time I was writhing on the floor and it was an emergency. I was rushed to hospital, where they removed the pregnancy and my right tube, which had ruptured.

So I was then back to square one. The cervical dysplasia was still there and this time I went to see a specialist who did a colposcopy, which should have been done before any surgery, and he said that it was so mild that nothing needed to be done at all and that I could try for a baby. I was so relieved! I started talking Clomid again, but after six or seven months I was still not pregnant. I really started feeling uncomfortable about taking it for so long.

I changed doctors and had more tests and it was clear that I still was not ovulating. I thought I should have a break for six months and try again. This time I took Clomid and had blood tests and a scan, which showed that I was ovulating properly but always on the ovary on my right, where there was no tube. This meant that the sperm could not reach the egg, unless in a one-in-a-million chance the tube on the other side picked it up.

This happened seven months in a row, which the doctor said was really unusual: although you do not ovulate from each ovary in turn, you normally expect some variation.

By then I was feeling that I was not ready for IVF but wondering what else I could do. I started going to a weekly workshop for women suffering fertility problems run by a wonderful therapist, who was in the same situation. It was really very helpful and saved me from going insane. I met women in the same situation and it prevented me from feeling like an outcast.

Then I had a hysterosalpingogram and the radiologist who did the X ray said that my only tube was fine. Next I saw the fertility specialist who had requested this test. He looked at the X ray and, without looking me in the eyes, said, "Tubal surgery or IVF?" A typical scientist—he didn't care about my feelings, I was just a number for him. I was shocked, so shocked and said, trying not to cry, that the radiologist had told me that the X ray showed my tube was fine. He asked me if I could read X rays and when I said no, he said "Your tube is not good. There are adhesions. Tubal surgery or IVF?" I asked what he would do, and he said it was my decision. I insisted and said he was the specialist. So he finally answered that he would go for tubal surgery and try to repair my tube (even though he couldn't be sure that this was possible until he had done a laparoscopy to see inside) so that I would have a small chance of getting pregnant naturally. He added that he would also try IVF after a few months. I knew the specialist was very good at tubal surgery, but he was so cold and uncaring that I couldn't contemplate having him near my body.

At around this time, I went to India with friends. Among the group was a woman who was a healer. I talked to her and mentioned that I was thinking of having tubal surgery. She said, "Don't have it—I have helped friends of mine and I'll try to help you." When we got home I went to see her and the first time she said I had blocked energy around the ovary on my left side, which was the side with the intact tube. This made sense because by then it seemed as if I had not been ovulating for a long time on that side.

I found it amazing that she could pick this up, so I went back to her for treatment on five consecutive days for half an hour each time. She used to put her hands over my ovaries and womb, where I would feel warmth and one time even a very light tingling sensation as if something was moving inside. She also laid her hands at the back of my neck, where the pituitary gland which controls the hormone production is. All the time she was reassuring me that my body was strong, that it would be fine. I went back the following month just before ovulation time. She asked me to take my temperature just to check that her treatment was helping me to ovulate. After a few days I stopped doing it as the temperature didn't seem to go up and it depressed me. But that month I became pregnant.

I thought it was amazing. By then it was two and a half years since the ectopic pregnancy and I had been taking Clomid on and off all that time. Sadly, when I got to my twelve-week scan the embryo had died. We had seen the heartbeat at eight weeks and nobody knew what had happened, but it was a missed abortion at around ten or eleven weeks. It was awful, really pretty hard and I felt I couldn't go on hoping that one day I would have a baby. Everything always seemed to go wrong.

I went back to see the healer two months later for a few sessions, but nothing happened. The following month I went again just before ovulation time and that time I became and stayed pregnant, until I had my son in August 1996. I really found it quite amazing that she could help so much on the physical side—it was proper healing, not faith healing. It was brilliant. She was very, very good.

At about the same time I started going to the healer, I found out about a fantastic program for women and men experiencing fertility problems. I was beginning to be a total wreck emotionally, and as I had always believed in the mind-body connection, I was convinced that doing some constructive work on the psychological side could only help me. I started to work with one of the founders of this program, a brilliant medical psychologist and hypnotherapist, and a very nice and caring woman. She worked on different levels, first by teaching me deep relaxation so that my body could have a break and heal, and then using regression techniques so that psychological blocks could be addressed. They have found that women experiencing fertility problems can have blocks which can prevent them from getting pregnant. They may only be simple, not necessarily anything like a big trauma. It could be that your work or career is very important to you, or that you might be afraid of getting pregnant, or scared of childbirth. Then the therapist helped me "reprogram" my mind so that my whole attitude towards pregnancy became positive and I finally believed it could happen, that I could get pregnant.

My husband, who was always very supportive and very open-minded, also went to see her a few times. He was always much more positive than me but after so many things going wrong, he was really interested in having some sessions. He thought it was great and not only for the fertility issue. The work with this therapist was so helpful to me that when I was pregnant I continued to see her, as getting pregnant was one thing but I wanted to be sure of carrying the pregnancy to full term. She also prepared me for childbirth, which really helped. I had a wonderful eight-hour labor with no pain relief; the baby was never in any distress and he has been a very contented and relaxed baby right from the birth.

During the whole pregnancy I was followed by a fertility consultant. I had finally found a really good and caring doctor who always listened to me. He put me on 75 mg aspirin a day from the seventh week of the pregnancy until three weeks before my baby's birth. It seems that one possible cause of miscarriage is blood clots and the aspirin keeping the blood fluid helps reduce the risk of miscarriage. He also gave me progesterone injections from the eighth week until the twelfth week, because this is a critical time for miscarriage. During this time the embryo can be a little late to take over the progesterone production from the corpus luteum. But I was the one who came up with the aspirin idea, as after the missed abortion I had informed myself very well about what could be done to prevent it from happening again. We really did collaborate in a way; I was also in charge of what was happening to my body.

I tried a lot of things to have my baby. I was very dedicated and in a way it was my project. I must say that the main things that helped me were the healing, the hypnotherapy, and having a supportive doctor. Going to a support group and sharing experiences with other women was also very helpful.

I believe that you have to be guided by what you feel is right for you. You have to go along your own path. You have to inform yourself very well so that you can find out about medical treatment and alternative therapies. Some women are happy with IVF; they feel ready for it and it goes well for them. Others are rushed into it, without being properly investigated or given any information about alternative ways. They might go through it and find it fails, feel awful and then start thinking how else they could help themselves, really doing it all backwards, which is physically and emotionally even more difficult.

Finding the right alternative therapists is very important. Lots of them can mean well, they are generally always caring and supportive but they are not always as qualified, gifted, and professional as the ones I have been lucky to find. I always left them feeling more positive, which is so important, because at some point you do need to believe that it can happen, that you can get pregnant, not only on a conscious level but also on a deeper level. But when I did the round of the fertility specialists I would come away feeling depressed. Of course, part of their job was to find what was wrong with me, so it made me feel even more pessimistic.

You have to inform yourself and decide with your doctor what tests you need and make sure that they are done. You should always keep some control over what is being done to your body and always be able to discuss it with your doctor. Unfortunately, some fertility specialists feel they do not have to listen to you and you do not dare challenge them. I believe that IVF is a very aggressive fertility treatment that should be done only after the couple's problems have been properly investigated, and as a last resort. It does seem that women are not looked at in a holistic way, so that something elementary can be overlooked. I was not checked for chlamydia after the ectopic pregnancy, when it is known that the infection can damage the tubes, therefore increasing the risk of ectopic pregnancy. I only found out later and was then prescribed a simple course of antibiotics. A friend of mine had to have three miscarriages before she was investigated more seriously and she had to ask for it. She was found to have a lupus condition that might have been treated by taking baby aspirin.

It is such a complex subject; there are so many physical and psychological factors which may cause fertility problems that it can be very difficult to treat. The classical medical approach is not always enough and you might have to try more than one alternative therapy. How can you treat the woman's body separately from her mind? Everybody agrees that a positive attitude will help a patient to heal faster and better; with fertility problems this is even more true. A person's emotions and feelings should never be neglected. It is really a shame that the medical profession is not more open to alternative approaches, as they could work together and create a wonderful synergy. I really wish that you could go to one place where different approaches were available and where someone knowledgeable could offer you advice and counseling so that some precious years would not be wasted.

· *Reflexology* ·

Reflexology, sometimes known as reflex zone therapy, seems to have a particularly good record in treating infertility, especially in women, although it can be useful for both partners, particularly when stress is a factor.

Reflexology is part of an ancient system of medicine that has been identified and reintroduced in this century. It reflects the belief that applying pressure on one part of the body can effect changes in another part, and so has its origins in the same philosophy as acupuncture, acupressure, and shiatsu. The idea is that each part of your body is reflected on a part of your feet and that ill health or disturbance of any particular part of your body can be detected in the corresponding part of your foot. Gentle and safe massage of the foot, concentrating on areas where disturbance is apparent, can assist the body to heal itself. Foot massage was used in China in the fourth century and was also practiced in Egypt, Japan, and by Native Americans for thousands of years.

Although it will depend on your situation, most reflexologists will treat you for six to eight sessions to begin with, each lasting an hour or more, at a rate of one or two sessions a week, gradually increasing the intervals as your health is restored.

The treatment itself is gentle and soothing and involves lying back while your feet are individually and thoroughly massaged, using the thumbs, with attention paid to each area. The areas which require special attention may be apparent to the reflexologist from the appearance of your feet and toes, or they may realize from your response where they are sensitive. Some people find the treatment painful, but experienced reflexologists believe that there is no need to exert strong pressure and that equally good results may be obtained by gentle massage.

The scope of reflexology is considerable, and although reflexologists would not claim to be able to cure serious diseases like cancer or multiple sclerosis, it can have impressive results in improving other conditions. It can relieve acute and chronic conditions including back pain, allergies, sinusitis, insomnia, constipation, migraine, and asthma. It is very good at treating menstrual problems: one practitioner states that painful periods are completely unnecessary and, as the stories below show, it has succeeded in treating apparently untreatable infertility in women.

Following reflexology treatment, the body may react quite strongly. It is possible for an illness briefly to become worse, or skin rashes to erupt. There may be changes in bowel action, increased urine output, extra vaginal discharge, mucus in the chest or nose, or an alteration in the menstrual cycle. Once the healing crisis is past, the body normally starts to recover and a big improvement in symptoms and skin type and texture may be seen. Reflexology is said to reduce the craving for chocolate experienced by many women.

Although reflexology is a good treatment for children, it is not generally recommended for use in the first three months of pregnancy, as there is a theoretical risk that it may cause miscarriage. After fourteen weeks, however, it can be very beneficial, to encourage relaxation and relieve the aches and pains of pregnancy. It is a good treatment for constipation, hemorrhoids, backache, swelling, heartburn and cystitis, and can be helpful for nausea and vomiting that continues after the first trimester. It can help pregnant women to sleep and may be used as pain relief in labor, encouraging contractions or even stimulating them when labor fails to start naturally.

There is little evidence on the efficacy of reflexology as an infertility treatment. However, a small trial in Denmark[12] which recruited women with fertility problems via a newspaper ad had some interesting results. In all, 108 women started treatment. The average length of time that they had been trying to conceive was 6.7 years and their average age was 30.2 years. They were offered free treatment consisting of sixteen reflexology sessions over seven to eight months, twice a week for the first month and then twice before each ovulation. The aim was to regulate menstruation, improve gastrointestinal function and liquid balance, and improve the quality of mucous membranes. The women were also invited to a lecture on diet and the use of vitamins and minerals. A large proportion dropped out, apparently because they had had a change of partner and no longer wanted to become pregnant. Of the remaining 61, 19 became pregnant within the first six months and 75 percent of the total experienced an improvement in muscle tensions, psychic imbalances, indigestion and circulation, and an enhancement of their general well-being.

· *Kim and Neil* ·

My husband and I had been trying for a baby for two to three years and, after suffering severe abdominal pains for seven months, I insisted that my GP refer me for a laparoscopy to investigate the cause of these pains and at the same time investigate the cause of my infertility.

He refused to do so, although due to the health insurance that I held with my employers, he eventually agreed to refer me privately. The laparoscopy carried out in February 1996 revealed the cause of my pain to be endometriosis and the cause of my infertility to be blocked tubes. The consultant advised us that IVF or adoption were really our only options for becoming parents.

My husband and I looked into IVF and were due to start our first attempt in May 1996. However, problems with my cycle kept delaying this and during this delay we came to the decision of not proceeding with IVF, because of the fear that we would end up heavily in debt and unable to get off the "merry-go-round," should the first attempt not work.

During this time I had been seeing a reflexologist to help with the stress and hopefully with the pain of endometriosis. I wasn't happy with taking painkillers for the foreseeable future, as pre- scribed by my GP. I continued to see my reflexologist once a week while my husband and I looked into the possibility of adoption.

At the end of June 1996 we experienced our little miracle when I was found to be pregnant. The doctor felt that with my medical problems this would be ectopic, but against all the odds a scan revealed a perfectly normal pregnancy at a stage of six weeks.

There was no doubt in my mind that reflexology had played a major part in this. I have continued to have reflexology throughout my pregnancy and have been extremely fit and well. Our baby is due any day now and you can imagine how excited my husband is at the thought of holding our own baby, conceived against all the odds.

Kim gave birth to Lauren, 7 lb 6 oz, after an eight-hour labor.

· *Judith* ·

I first went to see a reflexologist because I had a bad back, with lower-back stiffness and aching. I had tried an osteopath which hadn't helped, and this reflexologist had cured a friend of mine's bad shoulder, so I thought I would give it a try.

We had a happy, healthy eleven-year-old son and had been try- ing for another baby for four years. I had always had irregular periods, with gaps of two to four months between them; in fact, I had never known a 28-day cycle. Eventually I went to my doctor, who referred me to a professor of endocrinology at a large hospital.

He gave me a pelvic scan and blood tests which confirmed my doctor's suspicion that I had polycystic ovaries. The professor said it would probably not be a problem if I took Clomid. However, when I went back to my GP, the endocrinologist had written to him saying that for some reason my hormonal tests were not right, which meant that I was not eligible to take Clomid and that I should have a wedge resection of my ovaries instead.

I talked about it with my husband and we didn't really like it. Although I am a nurse I hate having any treatment myself, so we decided to leave it up to fate and whatever would be, would be.

I went to see the reflexologist, who took a full medical history and mentioned that the treatment could make periods regular. I was very sceptical about that, but the next day my period started without any of the symptoms of PMS that I usually got.

For the next couple of months my periods came in a regular cycle. Then last year I didn't have a period. I felt very low and depressed and had a lot of breast tenderness. I was expecting a period to start at any time, but it didn't. I was considering going to the GP about my symptoms and was just lying on the sofa feeling sorry for myself, when I was overcome by a wave of nausea and it suddenly occurred to me that I could possibly be pregnant. I thought that I had better make sure before taking anything that the doctor might prescribe and went out to get a pregnancy test, really resenting the the cost of it.

To my utter astonishment, it was positive. I went back to the reflexologist a couple of times during pregnancy, but I really didn't feel the need to go that often because, although I felt awfully sick to start with for 90 percent of the time, once I was past that I was really healthy. I had so much energy that I felt far healthier than I did normally and a lot better than in my previous pregnancy.

I had an appalling eighteen-hour labor because the baby was back to front, but two hours after she was born I felt as if I could run a marathon.

I can only pin it to the reflexology: we hadn't used contraception for years. I felt as if I had been out of kilter. She just gave me the tap and it all jumped back into place. I've got great faith in reflexology.

· *Melanie* ·

Almost every woman I knew was either pregnant or had just had a baby. I had hoped it would happen to me four years ago, but the months sailed by and, despite the amount of money I was spending on pregnancy-testing kits, the results were always negative.

I was 27 when we first thought about having a child. I had never imagined that there would be any problem. I'm a freelance publicist and Phil, my husband, is an architect. We share an office in our home and had looked forward to having a child and sharing the child care between us. We were not in any particular rush and initially I was very relaxed when we realized that I was not going to get pregnant immediately.

After a year I started to get a little anxious and arranged an appointment to have a chat with my GP. I was told that a year was not a long time to wait to have a child and was quoted the statistic that one couple in ten had difficulties conceiving. However, it was suggested that we had the initial non-invasive tests to see if there were any obvious problems which could be sorted out. We went ahead with these tests, which included a blood test for me, to look at hormone levels, and a sperm test for Phil, to check both his sperm count and sperm motility.

The results came back normal and we were faced with choosing between taking further medical action or waiting a little longer. It became very clear to us that if we were referred to a gynecologist we would be obliged to have a series of infertility tests—there was no question of having selective tests and we would be at the mercy of the medical profession. We had been interested in just having the postcoital test, and also in checking that my fallopian tubes were viable, but could not find a gynecologist willing to carry out only these tests. We did not want to go as far as having a laparoscopy, as we felt this was far too invasive and the control would disappear fast.

We soon realized that, although having a child was very important to us, if it was not going to happen naturally we would need to start to come to terms with childlessness. If the crunch came we knew we were not prepared to have IVF or similar infertility programs and felt that our lifestyle was far too selfish to consider adoption.

But after another year had passed I became quite desperate to have a child and found it difficult to spend time with families with young children. Everywhere I went women seemed to be pushing strollers and every shop seemed to be full of baby clothes.

I wanted to do something constructive to better my chances of conceiving that did not involve medical intervention. I started reading books about infertility and coping with childlessness and then came across a book called Natural Mothering *[see Further Reading]*. The book was aimed primarily at women who were pregnant and took a refreshing look at alternative medicines, including homeopathy, acupuncture, and osteopathy as ways of helping pregnancy and childbirth.

Included in the book was a short chapter on alternative ways of dealing with infertility and a couple of interesting case studies about women who had virtually given up hope but had conceived with the help of alternative therapies. I had never thought about alternative treatments, but now I could think of nothing else.

I had to decide which of the many alternative treatments would be best for me. Phil was very supportive and together we visited an acupuncturist and a reflexologist and after careful consideration opted for a course of reflexology. I had nothing to lose and although my reflexologist had never treated anyone for infertility, he had colleagues who had, and the success rate had been good.

The reflexologist works by applying a measured amount of pressure to different parts of the foot and depending on the patient's response at each stage, the practitioner works to restore the balance. Imbalances in the feet can be corrected by working on the painful areas and hence releasing blockages and restoring the flow of energy throughout the whole body. The feet play an important part in diagnosing problems and providing therapeutic treatment. Reflexology is used to help a variety of disorders, including many women's problems like premenstrual tension, period pains and menopause.

I was apprehensive about the treatment as the concept felt completely foreign, but in theory it made sense and I believed that reflexology would help me. My initial sessions showed that I had an underactive uterus—a lack of energy in the reproductive system. Each time the area relating to my uterus was touched on my foot, I squealed with pain. At home, when I tried to press the affected area and create the same pain I felt nothing.

As the treatment progressed this severe pain slowly subsided and I started to feel healthier and more aware of my body. The sessions also revealed that I was producing a lot of acid, so I changed my diet and reduced my acid intake avoiding citrus fruits, fizzy drinks, and any processed foods with high acid contents.

I had a reflexology session every week for six months, then every two weeks for three months. Each session lasted for an hour. Apart from feeling that I was doing something positive, I also seemed to cope better with the monthly arrival of my period. Being able to talk to someone outside my life on a regular basis about my fears and how I could cope with being surrounded by pregnant women and young babies made me feel less bitter and twisted. Phil also had a session to check that his body was functioning properly and to help him understand the changes that were taking place in my body.

During the tenth month of treatment my period was late. This had happened in the past, so I tried not to pay too much attention. But my feet were not giving any indications of a period about to start (my ankles usually started to throb before the onset of a period). However, after ten days I started to wonder if I might be pregnant and plucked up the courage to buy a pregnancy-testing kit and go through that very familiar procedure. This time there was no mistake: the result was positive. I was pregnant.

During the pregnancy I stopped my reflexology treatment—in the early months this is recommended to avoid miscarriage—as I felt my body had enough to deal with. I had a very healthy pregnancy and on January 6, 1993 (three days early) I gave birth to our baby daughter, Hannah Louise, weighing just 6 lb 1 oz. She was our reflexology baby. I had a straightforward delivery and survived a fifteen-hour labor with the use of only a Tens machine, which was very comforting.

Since having Hannah, I have heard of a case of a woman who used reflexology successfully to conceive a second child after being diagnosed as having blocked fallopian tubes. I am sure there are many more such success stories.

· *Relaxation* ·

A relaxed attitude to the problems of infertility is evidently helpful but may be increasingly hard to achieve. There has been furious debate (supported by research on either side) as to whether stress causes infertility or vice versa, but there is no doubt that the fact of not being able to have a child when you want one is inherently stressful, and so are the diagnostic tests and treatment, particularly the more invasive types.

Some of the measurable effects of stress are an increase in prolactin levels and a reduction in sperm quality (see pages 45, 101). Stress hormones such as catecholamines (adrenalin, nonadrenalin and dopamine) can affect the hypothalamus, pituitary gland, and reproductive organs by interacting with the hormones responsible. In normal ovulatory cycles, these are the gonadotropin-releasing hormones: prolactin, luteinizing hormone, and follicle-stimulating hormone. Endogenous opiates and melatonin secretion are altered by stress and interfere with ovulation.[13] One study[14] showed that up to 25 percent of the women subjects who were ovulating regularly and started treatment by artificial insemination by donor turned to an anovulatory state for a few months. The only reason that could be found was the stress of the treatment.

However, it is possible to relieve stress and encourage relaxation. In a trial which involved teaching fifteen couples autogenic training, a system of simple mental exercises designed to diminish stress and encourage relaxation, the authors found that the technique decreased prolactin levels in the women and reduced anxiety levels in both partners.[15] Of the fifteen couples who had had unexplained infertility for two or more years, the women were initially more prone to anxieties and likely to be introverted and feel tense and guilty. The training helped them to become less self-reproaching and one woman became pregnant. In this case the training involved gentle exercises in body awareness and physical relaxation, progressively involving the limbs, heart and circulation, lungs, and central nervous system. The couples were taught passive concentration and learned to practice it at will, so that they were able to control excessive stress whenever they wanted. They had eight sessions of an hour per week and were encouraged to practice at home for a few minutes three times a day.

All of the alternative therapies mentioned in this book will help you to deal with stress and encourage relaxation. Some, such as hypnotherapy or reflexology, may be particularly beneficial. If you wish to learn relaxation techniques you might find it easier to start by attending a course in one of the methods or philosophies that are available. It could be meditation, yoga or self-hypnosis. It is quite possible to teach yourself autogenic training, from a book, by means of a tape or by using a biofeedback machine. A method of autogenic training can be found in *Centering—A Guide to Inner Growth* by Sanders G. Laurie and Melvin J. Tucker (see Further Reading).

A brief example of what is involved in a simple relaxation technique is as follows:

Find a comfortable position where you will be warm and free from distractions. Starting with your toes and working upwards, become aware of any tensions in your body and let them go. Focus on your feet, ankles, calves, thighs, pelvis, stomach, chest, shoulders, arms, head, neck, face, jaw, mouth and scalp in turn. (When you first practice this technique you may find it easier to relax if you tense each set of muscles for ten seconds before letting go.) Become aware of how these muscles feel when they are relaxed and take three slow breaths before moving on to the next group. You should allow your breathing to become slow and deep, concentrating on the outward breath.

As you become more relaxed you will feel warmer, softer, and heavier. If you are distracted by extraneous thoughts, concentrate on images that you find pleasing—imagine that you are relaxing on a sunny beach or in a beautiful garden on a sunny day, or try to fill your whole mind and mind's eye with your favorite color.

7

BECOMING PREGNANT

Many people would like to believe that once a couple achieves a pregnancy after trying to conceive for a long time, the struggle is over. In some ways this is true; it is a terrific achievement and one of which to be proud. However, the legacy of a period of infertility, combined with anxiety about the pregnancy as well as other factors, may mean that it is not necessarily the time of unrestrained joy that may have been anticipated.

First, there are worries about the pregnancy. Couples who have had fertility problems are in some ways similar to those who have experienced miscarriage. Their assurance that everything will go well has gone forever. Their bodies have not functioned as they hoped and expected they would, and they may still regard themselves as infertile, with all the feelings of guilt, shame, defectiveness, and self-blame that this can entail.

If the woman has distanced herself from women with children, she may find herself quite isolated when she becomes pregnant. She no longer fits into the infertile category—and may not be welcomed by other infertile women—and may also feel that she does not fit into the fertile group, either. She may find that she is surprisingly ambivalent about being pregnant, understandably happy, yet somewhat dismayed as well.

It is quite normal to feel a bit trapped by pregnancy, in any circumstances, because your horizons automatically narrow and your life necessarily becomes more restricted, with the due date making the future finite. You may feel quite ill, too, and perhaps worried about the future or about how you will cope with labor or becoming a parent.

Some couples find it hard to tell their infertile friends that they are expecting a baby, as they know all too well how it might make them feel. Surprisingly, they may find it difficult to tell their fertile friends and their families, too, because of their concern over the baby. As a result of their previous experiences, they may be afraid to share their feelings of joy at all—even with each other—in case something goes wrong. Some pregnant women have felt more comfortable hiding their pregnancy and continuing their infertility support group.

Couples who have conceived with difficulty are often treated differently by prenatal staff. The pregnancy may be labeled "high-risk" and, although additional care may be welcome, it can also lead to unnecessary testing and intervention. Some women struggle to impress on staff that they want to be treated as if their pregnancy is a normal one, while doctors urge them to have an induction or cesarean section because it is a "precious" baby.

In one sense, the baby is at a higher risk of miscarriage. Miscarriage is much more common than is generally realized. Many of the women who have told their stories in this book have suffered miscarriages before finally having a baby. In one study,[1] 200 women who were planning to become pregnant and had no history of infertility were tested with sensitive pregnancy tests. It was found that there was a 31 percent miscarriage rate and a maximum pregnancy rate of 30 percent per cycle. Some of these pregnancies were very early, so the mothers may not have been aware of being pregnant, but these results give an idea of how common miscarriage can be. Unfortunately, there does seem to be a higher-than-average rate of miscarriage in women who have found it hard to conceive. This may be because the factor responsible for infertility also plays a part in maintaining pregnancy, but it is not clear why the majority of miscarriages occur. There are probably many different reasons.

Obviously, diet and lifestyle play a part: miscarriage rates are raised in those who smoke or drink or are poorly nourished. A miscarriage can be a devastating experience, although to outsiders it may not seem important, particularly if it happens in the early weeks. To the couple involved it means the loss of a much-wanted baby and it is hard to comprehend the depth of grief it can cause. It can take months to get over the experience and, in their anguish, many women feel that they are going crazy. Although little discussed, these feelings are normal and do lessen in time. Support for those who have lost a baby, and a publication entitled *Early Pregnancy Loss,* can be obtained through an organization called Women to Women (see Useful Addresses).

You may not be able to avoid miscarrying, but it is certainly important to look after yourself well in pregnancy. Don't push yourself too hard; if having a baby is the most important thing to you, treat it as such and take steps to accommodate the pregnancy into your life rather than carrying on as if you were not pregnant. If you have received help from a therapist in order to become pregnant, keep in touch with him or her during the pregnancy. The therapist may be able to treat you so that you have a healthy pregnancy and give birth to a healthy baby.

Try to enjoy the pregnancy, even if you are very fearful of losing the baby. You can take pleasure in it, and distancing yourself from your baby just in case you miscarry will not make it any easier if you do. With luck, it will be a time that you are able to remember fondly.

REFERENCES

Chapter 1

1. Downey J. Mood disorders, psychiatric symptoms and distress in women presenting for infertility evaluation. *Fertility and Sterility*, September 1989, vol. 52, no. 3, pp. 425–32.
2. Skakkabaek N., Giwercman A., de Krester D. Pathogenesis and management of male infertility. *Lancet*, 1994, vol. 343, pp. 1473–9.
3. Pryor J. Male infertility: drug therapy and surgical treatment. *Current Obstetrics and Gynaecology Opinion*, 1996, vol. 6, pp. 12–17.
4. Matorras R., Rodriguez F., Pijoan J. Are there any clinical signs and symptoms that are related to endometriosis in infertile women? *American Journal of Obstetrics and Gynecology,* vol. 174, no. 2, pp. 620–23.
5. Hughes E., Fedorkow D., Collin J. A quantitive overview of controlled trials in endometriosis-associated infertility. *Fertility and Sterility,* May 1993, vol. 59, no. 5, pp. 963–70.

Chapter 2

1. Jirka J., Schuett S., Foxall M. Loneliness and social support in infertile couples. *Journal of Obstetric, Gynecology and Neonatal Nursing,* January 1996, vol. 25, no. 1, pp. 55–60.
2. Schoener C., Krysa L. The comfort and discomfort of infertility. *Journal of Obstetrical, Gynecological and Neonatal Nursing,* February 1996, vol. 25, no. 2, pp. 167–72.
3. Lieberman B., Buck P., Hazledine C. Why women delay returning for the replacement of their frozen embryos. *Journal of the British Fertility Society (2) Human Reproduction 11,* 1996, National Supplement pp. 128–31.
4. Templeton A. Infertility—Epidemiology, aetiology, effective management. *Health Bulletin,* September 1995, vol. 53 (3), pp. 294–8.
5. *Sunday Times* (London), January 25, 1997, p. 10.
6. Unruh A., McGrath P. The psychology of female infertility: toward a new perspective. *Health Care for Women International,* 1985, vol. 6, pp. 369–81.
7. van Balen F., Trimbos-Kemper T. Involuntarily childless couples: their desire to have children and their motives. *Journal of Psychosomatic Obstetrics and Gynecology,* 1995, vol. 16, pp. 137–44.

8. van Balen F., Trimbos-Kemper T. J. Long-term infertile couples: a study of their well-being. *Psychosom. Obstet. Gynecol.*, 1993, Special Issue, pp. 53–60.

9. Zoeten M.J. *et al.* The motivations and expectations of women waiting for IVF. *Human Reproduction*, 1987, vol. 2, p. 623.

10. McWhinnie A. A study of parenting IVF and DI children. *Medicine and Law*, 1995, vol. 14, pp. 501–8.

11. Schoener, pp.167–172.

Chapter 3

1. Benshushan A., Shushan A., Pattiel O. Ovulation induction with clomiphene citrate. *European Journal of Obstetrics and Gynecology*, 1995, vol. 62, pp. 261–2.

2. Derman S., Adashi A. Induction of ovulation. *Comprehensive Therapy* 1995, vol. 21 (10), pp. 583–9.

3. Saunders D.M., Lancaster P.A.L., Redisich E.L. Increased pregnancy failure rates after clomiphene following assisted reproductive technology. *Human Reproduction*, 1992, vol. 7, pp. 1154–8.

4. Whittemore A.S., Harris R., Intyre J. The Collaborative Ovarian Cancer Group: characteristics relating to ovarian cancer risk; collaborative analysis of 12 U.S. case-control studies. Stage 2 invasive epithelial ovarian cancers in white women. *American Journal of Epidemiology*, 1992, vol. 136, pp. 1184–1203.

5. Rossing M.A., Dalling J., Weiss M.D., Moore D.M. Risk of breast cancer in a cohort of infertile women. *Gynecological Oncology*, vol. 60, pp. 3–7.
    See also
    Caro J.J., Johannes C.B., Hartz S.C. Characteristics relating to ovarian cancer risk: collaborative analysis risk of 12 U.S. case-control studies. Stage 2 invasive epithelial ovarian cancers in white women. *American Journal Epidemiology*, 1993, vol. 137, p. 928.
    Cohen J., Forman R., Harlap S. IFFS expert group report on the Whittemore study related to the risk of ovarian cancer associated with the use of infertility agents. *Human Reproduction*, 1993, vol. 8, pp. 996–9.
    Spiritas R., Kaufman S.C., Alexander N.J. Fertility drugs and ovarian cancer: red alert or red herring? *Fertility and Sterility*, 1993, vol. 59, pp. 291–3.
    Rossing M.A., Dalling J.R., Weiss N.S. Ovarian tumours in a cohort of infertile women. *New England Journal of Medicine*, 1994, vol. 331, pp. 771–6.
    Bristow R., Karlan B. Ovulation induction, infertility and ovarian cancer risk. *Fertility and Sterility*, October 1996, vol. 66, no. 4, pp. 496–507.
    Bristow R., Karlan B. The risk of ovarian cancer after treatment for infertility. *Current Opinion in Obstetrics and Gynecology*, 1996, vol. 8, pp. 32–7.

6. Werler M., Louik C., Shapiro S. Ovulation induction and risk of neural tube defects. *Lancet*, 1994, vol. 344, pp. 445–6.

7. Shaw G., Lammer E., Velic E. Ovulation induction by clomiphene and neural tube defects. Letter to the editor, *Reproductive Toxicology*, 1995, vol. 9, no. 4, pp. 399–40.

8. White L. *et al.* Neuroectodermal tumours in children born after assisted conception. *Sydney Lancet*, 1990, vol. 336, p. 1577, and Kobayashi N *et al.* Childhood neuroectodermal tumours and malignant lymphoma after maternal ovulation induction. Tokyo *Lancet* (letter), 1990, vol. 336, p. 1577.

9. LaBella F.S., Brandes L.J. Enhancement of tumor growth by drugs with some common molecular actions. *Molecular Carcinogenesis*, 1996, vol. 16, pp. 68–76.

10. Michalek A., Buck G., Wasca P., Freedman P. *et al.* Gravid health status, medication use and risk of neuroblastoma. *American Journal of Epidemiology*, vol. 143, pp. 996–1001.

11. Golan A., Ron-El R., Herman A., Soffer Y. Ovarian hyperstimulation syndrome: an update review. *Obstetrics and Gynecology Surveillance*, vol. 44, pp. 430–40.

12. Bar-Hara I., Orvieto R., Dicker D., Dekel A. *et al.* A severe case of ovarian hyperstimulation syndrome: 65 liters of ascites aspirated in an on-going IVF-ET twin pregnancy. *Gynecology and Endocrinology*, 1995, vol. 9, pp. 295–8.

13. Derman and Adashi, pp. 583–9.

14. Asch R., Lo H., Balmaceda J., Weckstein L. Severe ovarian hyperstimulation syndrome in assisted reproductive technology: definition of high-risk groups. *Human Reproduction*, vol. 6, pp. 1395–9.

15. Collins J. A. and Hughes E.G. Pharmocological interventions for the induction of ovulation. *Drugs*, Sept 1995, 50 (3) pp. 480–94.

16. Dawood Y. In vitro fertilisation, gamete intrafallopian transfer and super-ovuation with intrauterine insemination: Efficacy and potential health hazards on babies delivered. *American Journal of Obstetrics and Gynecology*, vol. 174, no. 4, pp. 1208–17.

17. Luke B., Keith L. The contribution of singletons, twins and triplets to low birth weight, infant mortality and handicap in the United States. *Journal of Reproductive Medicine*, 1992, vol. 37, pp. 661–6.

18. Collins and Hughes, 480–94.

19. Derman and Adashi, pp. 583–9.

20. Collins and Hughes, pp. 480–94.

21. Soules M.R. Now that we have painted ourselves into a corner. *Fertility and Sterility*, November 1996, vol. 66, no. 5.

22. Dawood, pp. 1208–17.

23. Gleicher N., Vander Laan B., Pratt D. Background pregnancy rates in an infertile population. *Human Reproduction*, 1996, vol. 11, no. 5, pp. 1011–12.
See also
Collins J.A., Burrows E.A., Willan A.R. The prognosis for live birth among untreated infertile couples. *Fertility and Sterility*, vol. 64, pp. 22–8.

24. Dawood, pp. 1208–17.
25. Wang J.X., Clark A.M., Kirby L.A. The obstetric outcome of singleton pregnancies following in vitro fertilization and gamete intra-fallopian transfer. *Human Reproduction*, 1994, vol. 9, pp. 141–6. Tanbo T., Dale P.O., Lunde O., Moe N. Obstetric outcome in singleton pregnancies after assisted conception. *Human Reproduction*, 1995, vol. 86, pp. 188–92.
26. Dawood, pp. 1208–17.
27. Lancaster P. Assisted conception: Health Services and Evaluators. *International Journal of Technology Assessment in Health Care*, 1991, vol. 7, no. 4, pp. 485–99.
28. Deaton J.L., Gibson M., Blackmer K.M. A randomized trial of clomiphene citrate and intrauterine insemination in couples with unexplained infertility or surgically corrected endometriosis. *Fertility and Sterility*, 1986, vol. 46, pp. 135–7.

Fisch P., Casper R.F., Brown S.E. Unexplained infertility: evaluation of treatment with clomiphene citrate and human chorionic gonadotropin. *Fertility and Sterility*, 1989, vol. 51, pp. 828–33.

Glazener C. M. A., Coulson C., Lambert P. M. Clomiphene treatment for women with unexplained infertility: placebo-controlled study of hormonal responses and conception rates. *Gynecology and Endocrinology*, 1990, vol. 4, pp. 75–83.

Chapter 4

1. Meyers M., Weinshel M., Scharf C. An infertility primer for family therapists: 11. working with couples who struggle with infertility. *Family Process*, June 1995, vol. 34.

Chapter 5

1. Stanton C., Gray R. Effects of caffeine consumption on delayed conception. *American Journal of Epidemiology*, 1995, vol. 142, no. 12, pp. 1322–9.
2. Wilcox A., Weinberg C., Baird D. Caffeinated beverage and decreased fertility. *Lancet*, 1988, vol. 2, pp. 1453–5.
3. Dluglosz I., Bracken M. Reproductive effects of caffeine: a review and theoretical analysis. *Epidemiology Review*, 1992, vol. 14, pp. 83–100. Eskenazi B. Caffeine during pregnancy: grounds for concern? *Journal of the American Medical Association*, 1993, vol. 270, pp. 2973–4. Infant-Rivard C., Fernandez A., Gauthier R. Fetal loss associated with caffeine intake before and during pregnancy. *Journal of the American Medical Association*, 1993, vol. 270, pp. 2940–43.
4. Lane J., Steege J., Rupp S. Menstrual cycle effects on caffeine elimination in the human female. *European Journal of Clinical Pharmacology*, 1992, vol. 43, pp. 543–6.
5. Scott R., MacPherson A., Yates R.W.S. Selenium supplementation in subfertile human males. In: Fischer P.W.F., L'Abbe M. R., Cockell K.A.,

Gibsom R.S. (eds). Trace Elements in man and animals—9 (TEMA 9). Ottawa NRC Research Press, 1997.

6. Rayman M. Dietary selenium: time to act. *British Medical Journal*, February 1997, vol. 3148, pp. 387–8.

7. Aitken R.J., Clarkson J.S., Hargreave J.B., Wu F.C.W., Analysis of the relationship between defective sperm function and the generation of reactive oxygen species in cases of oligozoospermia. *J. Androl.*, 1989, vol. 10, pp. 214–20.

8. Miscarriage Association Newsletter, 1992.

9. Clark A., Ledger W., Gallethy C. Weight loss results in significant improvement in pregnancy and ovulating rates in anovulatory obese women. *Human Reproduction*, vol. 10, pp. 2705–27.

10. Barbieri R.L., Smith S., Ryan K.J. The role of hyperinsulinaemia in the pathogenisis of ovarian hyperadrogenism. *Fertility and Sterility*, 1988, vol. 50, pp. 197–212. Dunaif A. Do androgenes directly regulate gonadotropin secretion in the polycystic ovary syndrome? *Journal of Clinical Endocrinology and Metabolism*, 1988, vol. 63, pp. 215–221. Pasquali R. and Casimiri F. The impact of obesity on hyperandrogenism and polycystic ovary syndrome in premenopausal women. *Clinical Endocrinology* (Oxford), 1993, pp. 1–16.

11. van der Spuy A.M., Steer P.J., McCusker M. Outcome of pregnancy in underweight women after spontaneous and induced ovulation. *British Medical Journal*, 296, pp. 962–5.

12. Doyle W., Crawford M.A., Wynn A.H.A., Wynn S.W. The association between maternal diet and birth dimensions. *Journal of Nutritional Medicine*, 1990, vol. 1, pp. 9–17.

13. *New Generation*. March 1994, vol. 13, no.1, pp 6–7.

14. Athanasiou S. *et al.* Effect of indomethacin on follicular structure, vascularity and function over the periovulatory period in women. *Fertility and Sterility*, March 1996, vol. 65, no. 3.

15. Judy Priest. *Drugs in Conception, Pregnancy and Childbirth* (HarperCollins, 1996).

16. Powell P., Murdoch H.T. Anabolic steroid abuse body builders and male subfertility. Lloyd F.H., *British Medical Journal*, July 1996, vol. 313, pp. 100–101.

17. Turek P.J., Williams R.H., Gilbaugh J.H. The reversibility of anabolic steroid-induced azoospermia. *J. Urology*, 1995, vol. 153, pp. 1628–30. Anabolic steroid induced hypogonadotrophic hypogonadism. *American Journal of Sports Medicine*. 1990, vol. 18, pp. 229–310.

18. Ravenholt R.T. Cell to organism: Tobacco's influence on development. In: Rosenburg M.J., *Smoking and Reproductive Health*. Littleton (MA) Year Book, Medical Publishers Inc., 1987, p. 10–16.

19. Hughes, E., Brennan B. Does cigarette smoking impair natural or assisted fecundity? *Fertility and Sterility*, November 1996, vol. 66, no. 5, pp. 679–89.

20. Band D. and Wilcox A. Cigarette smoking associated with delayed conception. *Journal of the American Medical Association*, 1985, vol. 253, pp. 2979–83.
21. Harrison K.L., Breen T.M., Hennessey J.F. The effect of patient smoking habit on the outcome of IVF and GIFT treatment. *Australia and New Zealand Journal of Obstetrics and Gynaecology*, 1990, vol. 30, pp. 340–4.
22. Thrupp L.A. Sterilisation of workers from pesticide exposure: the causes and consequences of DBCP-induced damage in Costa Rica and beyond. *International Journal of the Health Services*, 1991, vol. 21 (4), pp. 731–57.
23. de Cock J., Westveer K., Heederik D., te-Velde E. Time to pregnancy and occupational exposure to pesticides in fruit growers in the Netherlands. *Occupational and Environmental Medicine*, October 1994, vol. 51 (10), pp. 693–9.
24. Strohmer H., Boldizsar A., Plockinger B. Agricultural work and male infertility. *American Journal of Industrial Medicine*, November 1993 vol. 24 (5), pp. 587–92.
25. Gerhard I., Eckrich W., Runnebaum B. Toxic pollutants and fertility disorders: solvents and pesticides. *Geburtshilfe—Frauenheilkd*, March 1993, vol. 53 (3), pp. 147–60.
26. Bents H. Psychology of male infertility—a literature survey. *International Journal of Andrology*, 1985, vol. 8, pp. 325–336.
27. Giblin P.T., Ager J.W. *et al*. Effects of stress and characteristic adaptability on semen quality in healthy men. *Fertility and Sterility*, 1988, vol. 49, pp. 127–132.
28. Cui Ke-Hui. The effect of stress on semen reduction in the marmoset monkey. *Human Reproduction*, 1996, vol. 11, no. 3, pp. 568–73.
29. Rachootin P., Olsen J. The Risk of Fertility and Delayed Conception associated with exposures in the Danish Workplace. *Journal of Occupational Medicine*, vol. 25, no. 5, May 1983, pp. 394–402.

Chapter 6

1. Gerhard I., Postneek F. Auricular acupuncture in the treatment of female infertility. *Gynecological Endocrinology*, September 6, 1992, vol. 3, pp. 171–81.
2. The treatment of immunological infertility with Chinese medical herbs of ziyin jianghuo. *Chung-Kuo Chung Hsi i Chieh Ho Tsa Chih*, 1995, vol. 15 (1), pp. 3–5.
3. Yang X.F., Wci T., Tong J. Clinical and experimental study or composite wuzi dihuang liquor in treating male infertility. *Chung-Kuo Chung Hsi i Chieh Ho Tsa Chih*, 1995, vol. 15 (4), pp. 209–12.
4. Chen R.A., and Wen H. Clinical study on treatment of male infertility with shengjing pill. *Chung-Kuo Chung Hsi i Chieh Ho Tsa Chih*, 1995, vol. 15(4) pp. 205–8.

5. Ishikawa H., Manabe F., Zhangtao H. The hormonal response to HCG stimulation in patients with male infertility before and after treatment with Hochuekkito. *American Journal of Chinese Medicine*, 1992, vol. 20 (2), pp. 157–65.

6. Yu C.Q., Zhai M.F., Yao R.M. Effect of Nei-Yi recipe on plasma beta-endorphin levels during menstrual cycle in women with endometriosis. *Chung-Kuo Chung Hsi i Chieh Ho Tsa Chih*, 1995, vol. 15, (1) pp, 6–8.

7. Gerhard I., Reimers G., Keller C., *et al.* Vergleich homeopathischer Einzelmittelmit konventioneller Hormontherapie. *Therapeutikon* July 1993. vol. 7(7/8) pp. 309–315.

8. Gerhard Von I., Keller C., Shmuck M., Wirksamkeit homoopathischer Einzel- und Komplexmittel bei Frauen mit unerfulltem Kinderwunsch. *Erfrahrungsheilkunde*, vol.3, pp. 132–ff.

9. Gravitz M.A. Hypnosis in the treatment of functional infertility. *American Journal of Clinical Hypnosis*, July 1995, Vol. 38, 1, pp.22–6.

10. Mackett J., Maden W. Simple hypnotherapy for infertility. In Waxman D. *et al.*, *Hypnosis: The Fourth European Congress at Oxford*, pp. 201–5 (London, Whurr, 1989).

11. Leckie F.H., Further gynecological conditions treated by hypnotherapy. *The International Journal of Clinical and Experimental Hypnosis*, 1965, vol. 13, pp. 11–25. Also of interest Crasilneck H.B., and Hall J.A. *Clinical hypnosis: Principles and applications.* 2nd ed. (Orlando, Grune and Stratton, 1985.)

12. Leila Eriksen. *FDZ Journal*, 1990, Zoneterapeuten 5.

13. Schenker J., Meirow D., Schenker E. Stress and human reproduction. *European Journal of Obstetrics and Gynecology and Reproductive Biology*, 1992, vol. 45, pp. 1–8.

14. Glezerman M. Two hundred and seventy cases of artificial donor insemination: Management and results. *Fertility and Sterility*, 1981, vol. 35, pp. 180–87.

15. O'Moore A., O'Moore R., Harrison R. Psychosomatic aspects in idiopathic infertility: effects of treatment with autogenic training. *Journal of Psychosomatic Research*, 1993, vol. 27, no. 2, pp. 145–51.

Chapter 7

1. Zinaman M., Clegg E., Brown C. Estimated rates of human fertility and pregnancy loss. *Fertility and Sterility*, March 1996, vol. 65, no. 3.

FURTHER READING

Acupuncture

Acupressure Techniques—A Self-Help Guide, Julian Kenyon (Healing Arts Press, 1988).

Acupuncture Energetics—A Workbook for Diagnostics and Treatment, Mark Seem, Ph.D. (Healing Arts Press, 1991).

Path of Pregnancy, Bob Flaws (Paradigm Publications, 1983).

Aromatherapy

The Encyclopedia of Aromatherapy, Chrissie Wildwood (Healing Arts Press, 1996).

Aromatherapy for Women, Maggie Tisserand, (Healing Arts Press, 1996).

Aromatherapy for Mother and Baby, Allison England, R.N. (Healing Arts Press, 1994).

Chemicals

Human Ecology and Susceptibility to the Chemical Environment, Theron G. Randolph (Charles C. Thomas, 1981).

Safe Food: Eating Wisely in a Risky World, Michael Jacobson (Living Planet Press, 1991).

Chinese Herbal Medicine

Healing with Chinese Herbs, Richard Hyatt (Healing Arts Press, 1990).

Diet

Candida Albicans: Could Yeast be your Problem? Leon Chaitow (Healing Arts Press, 1998).

Food Allergies and Food Intolerance, Jonathan Brostoff and Linda Gamlin (Healing Arts Press, 1999).

The Healing Cuisine of China—300 Recipes for Vibrant Health and Longevity, Zhuo Zhao and George Ellis (Healing Arts Press, 1998).

Planning a Baby?, Sarah Brewer (Vermillion, 1996).

Drugs

The Complete Guide to Prescription and Nonprescription Drugs, H. Winter Griffith, M.D. (The Body Press/Perigee, 1999).

The PDR Family Guide to Prescription Drugs (Three Rivers Press, 1998).

Drugs in Conception, Pregnancy and Childbirth, Judy Priest, (HarperCollins, 1996).

Herbal medicine

The Herbal Handbook—A User's Guide to Medical Herbalism, David Hoffman (Healing Arts Press, 1998).

The Family Herbal, Barbara and Peter Theiss (Healing Arts Press, 1993).

Herbal Healing for Women, Rosemary Gladstar (Simon and Schuster, 1993).

The Male Herbal, Health Care for Men and Boys, (Crossing Press, 1991).

Homeopathy

Homeopathic Medicine for Women, Trevor Smith, M.D. (Healing Arts Press, 1989).

Medical Treatment of Infertility

Conceiving Your Baby: How Medicine Can Help, Sally Keble (Cedar, 1995).

Natural family planning

Healing Mind, Healthy Woman, Alice Domar, Ph.D. (Doubleday, 1997).

The Whole Person Fertility Program: A Revolutionary Mind-Body Process to Help You Conceive, Niravi Payne, M.S. (Three Rivers Press, 1998).

Taking Charge of Your Fertility: The Definitive Guide to Natural Birth Control and Pregnancy Achievement, Toni Weschler, M.P.M. (HarperCollins, 1995).

Nutrition

Prescription for Nutritional Healing, James F. Balch, M.D. and Phyllis A. Balch, C.M.C. (Avery Publishing Group, 1997).

Nutritional Medicine, Drs. Stephen Davies and Alan Stewart (Pan, 1987).

The Whole Food Bible, Chris Kilham (Healing Arts Press, 1997).

Whole Food Facts—The Complete Reference Guide, Evelyn Roehl (Healing Arts Press, 1996).

The New Laurel's Kitchen—A Handbook for Vegetarian Cookery and Nutrition, Laurel Robertson, Brian Ruppenthal, and Carol L. Flinders (Ten Speed Press, 1986).

Pregnancy

Natural Mothering—A Guide to Holistic Therapies for Pregnancy, Birth, and Early Childhood, Nicky Wesson (Healing Arts Press, 1997).

Positive Pregnancy Fitness, Sylvia Klein Olkin (Avery Publishing Group, 1987).

Energetic Pregnancy, Elizabeth Davis (Celestial Arts Press, 1995).

Reflexology

Reflex Zone Therapy of the Feet—A Textbook for Therapists, Hanne Marquardt, (Healing Arts Press, 1984).

The Reflexology Manual, Pauline Wills (Healing Arts Press, 1995).

Reflexology Today, Doreen E. Bayly (Healing Arts Press, 1988).

Relaxation

The Stress-Free Habit, John Perkins (Healing Arts Press, 1989).

Centering—A Guide to Inner Growth, Sanders G. Laurie and Melvin J. Tucker (Destiny Books, 1993). Audiocassette available as well.

An Herbal Guide to Stress Relief, David Hoffman (Healing Arts Press, 1991).

Women's Health

Alternative Health Care for Women, Patsy Westcott and Leyardia Black, N.D. (Healing Arts Press, 1988).

Women's Bodies, Women's Wisdom, Christiane Northrup, M.D. (Bantam Books, 1998).

USEFUL ADDRESSES

Alternative Therapies

American Association of Acupuncture
and Oriental Medicine
Tel: 610-266-1433
For referral to an acupuncturist
near you.

The Council of Colleges of
Acupuncture and Oriental
Medicine
8403 Colesville Road, Suite 370
Silver Springs, MD 20910
Tel: 301-608-9175
Web site: www.ccaom.org

The American Association of
Naturopathic Physicians
2366 Eastlake Avenue, Suite 322
Seattle, WA 98102
Tel: 206-298-0125
web site: www.naturopathic.org

The American Holistic Medical
Association/Foundation
2727 Fairview Avenue East
Seattle, WA 98102
Tel: 206-322-6842

Candida Research and Information
Foundation
P.O. Box JF
College Station, TX 77841
Tel: 409-694-8687
Send a SASE to the address above
for a free informational brochure.

American Herbal Products
Association (AHPA)
P.O. Box 2410
Austin, TX 78768

Herb Research Foundation
1007 Pearl Street, Suite 200
Boulder, CO 80302
Tel: 303-449-2265
Web site: www.herbs.org

Homeopathic Educational Services
2124 Kittredge Street
Berkeley, CA 94704
Tel: 510-649-0294
Web site: www.homeopathic.com

National Center for Homeopathy
801 N. Fairfax Street, Suite 306
Alexandria, VA 22314
Tel: 703-548-7790

American Council of Hypnotism
Examiners
312 Riverdale Drive
Glendale, CA 91204
Tel: 818-242-1159
Web site: www.gilboyne.com

Transformational Hypnotherapy
Ti Caine, C.H.T.
15446 Deerhorn Road
Sherman Oaks, CA 91403-4307
Tel: 818-995-0011

International Institute of Reflexology
P.O. Box 12642
St. Petersburg, FL 33733-2642

Yoga Journal
2054 University Avenue
Berkeley, CA 94704
The July/August edition includes a
national listing of yoga teachers.

Drugs and alcohol

Alcoholics Anonymous
475 Riverside Drive, 11th Floor
New York, NY 10115

National Clearinghouse for Alcohol
and Drug Information
11426-28 Rockville Pike, Suite 200
Rockville, MD 20847-2345
Tel: 800-729-6686 or 301-443-6500

National Institute on Alcohol Abuse
and Alcoholism
6000 Executive Boulevard Suite
Rockville, MD 20892-7003
Tel: 301-443-3860

National Institute on Drug Abuse
5600 Fishers Lane
Rockville, MD 20857
Tel: 310-443-6245

Do It Now Foundation
P. O. Box 27568
Tempe, AZ 85285-7568
Tel: 602-491-0393
Publishes substance abuse and
behavioral health information.

Endometriosis

Endometriosis Association
8585 North 76th Place
Milwaukee, WI 53223
Tel: 800-992-ENDO (United States)
    800-426-2END (Canada)
Web site: www.endometriosisassn.org

Infertility

American Society for Reproductive
    Medicine
1209 Montgomery Highway
Birmingham, AL 35216
Tel: 205-978-5000
Web site: www.asrm.org
E-mail: asrm@asrm.org

Fertility Research Foundation
1430 Second Avenue, Suite 103
New York, NY 10021
Tel: 212-744-5500
E-mail: frfbaby@msn.com

Alice Domar, Ph.D.
Mind/Body Medical Clinic
    Women's Center
Deaconess Hospital
Boston, MA 02215
Tel: 617-632-9530
Dr. Domar offers stress reduction
approaches that help women manage
the biochemical effects of stress,
including the stress associated with
fertility interventions. Tapes are also
available.

Niravi Payne, M.S.
Whole Person Fertility Program
100 Remsen Street
Brooklyn, NY 11201
Tel: 800-666-HEALTH or
    718-625-4801
E-mail: niravi@aol.com
Ms. Payne is a therapist who works with
the mind/body connection in women with
infertility. The pregnancy success rate of
her program is very high.

Marcelle Pick, R.N.C.
Women to Women
3 Marina Road
Yarmouth, ME 04096
Tel: 207-846-6163
Fax: 207-846-6167

Pregnancy

International Childbirth Education
   Association
P.O. Box 20048
Minneapolis, MN 55420
Tel: 612-854-8660

National Organization of Mothers of
   Twins Club
P.O. Box 23188
Albuquerque, NM 87192-1188
Tel: 800-243-2276
Web site: www.nomotc.org

Planned Parenthood Federation of
   America
810 Seventh Avenue
New York, NY 10019
Tel: 212-541-7800
Web site: www.plannedparenthood.org

Pregnancy loss

Perinatal Loss
2116 N.E. 18th Avenue
Portland, OR 97212
Tel: 503-284-7426
Fax: 503-282-8985

Women to Women
3 Marina Road
Yarmouth, ME 04096
Tel: 207-846-6163
Fax: 207-846-6167
Publication available through this
office entitled *Early Pregnancy Loss,*
by Bethany Hays, M.D.

Smoking

Nicotine Anonymous
P.O. Box 591777
San Francisco, CA 94159-1777
Tel: 415-750-0328
Web site: www.nicotine-anonymous.org

Sound Nutrition
Tel: 800-844-6645
Distributor of Sulfonil supplements
which can help curb cravings.

The Lenair Technique
75 Scotland Road
Newbury, MA 01951
Tel: 508-465-7711
A bioelectrical and electromagnetic
treatment for addictions. See also the
"Do It Now Foundation" entry under
"Drugs and alcohol," and the acupunc-
ture resources under "Alternative
therapies."

Other useful addresses

Aroma Vera Inc.
5901 Rodeo Road
Los Angeles, CA 90016-4312
Tel: 310-280-0407
Web site: www.aromavera.com
Essential oils from organically grown
plants.

Avena Botanicals
219 Mill Street
Rockport, ME 04858
Tel: 207-594-0694
Herbalist Deb Soule distributes
herbal remedies. Catalog available for
$2. Also available *The Roots of
Healing: A Woman's Book of Herbs.*

Center for Nuclear and Toxic Waste
   Management
Web site: www.cnwm.berkeley.edu
This Web site, run by the University
of California at Berkeley, provides
links to academic reports, government sites, and citizens' action groups
focusing on toxic waste.

Citizens for Health
P.O. Box 2260
Boulder, CO 80306
Tel: 800-357-2211 or
    303-417-0772
Fax: 303-417-9378
A national and international network
of people who want to exercise their
right to make informed choices
about their health care.

Feingold Association of the
   United States
P.O. Box 6550
Alexandria, VA 22306
Tel: 703-768-3287
Provides information on the effects
of food and food additives on health,
behavior, and learning.

Quality Life Herbs
P.O. Box 565
Yarmouth, ME 04096
Tel: 207-842-4929
Fax: 207-846-3168
International distributor of Chinese
herbs. Quality Life will fill written
prescriptions from licensed practitioners of Chinese medicine; they
recommend a full diagnostic consultation and caution against
self-diagnosis.

Uttati International
400 South Beverly Drive, Suite 214
Beverly Hills, CA 90212
Tel: 310-556-5717
Source of fine imported aroma-
therapy oils

GLOSSARY

Analogue (as in drugs)—similar to another drug or synthetic version of organic material.

Anencephaly—a neural tube defect which results in a fetus developing without a brain. It is incompatible with life.

Androgen—male hormones including testosterone. They are present in men and in smaller amounts in women. Androgen deficiency can be responsible for infertility.

Anovulation—failure of the egg to develop and be released from the ovary mid-cycle.

Atherosclerosis—disease of the arterial wall in which the layer thickens.

Auto-immune—a reaction of the body's immune system against the organs or tissues of his or her own body.

Azoospermia—sperm are completely absent.

Chlamydia trachomatis—a sexually transmitted disease which may result in salpingitis or inflammation of the fallopian tubes and consequent female infertility. The disease may cause symptoms of PID or no symptoms at all. In men it may cause discharge from the penis and swelling of testes and cause infertility if untreated.

Cytotoxic drugs—anticancer drugs.

Ectopic pregnancy—pregnancy which develops outside the uterus, most often in the fallopian tube but occasionally elsewhere in the pelvic cavity. Symptoms begin before 12 weeks of pregnancy and can include severe pain in the abdomen, and sometimes bleeding from the vagina. If the tube ruptures, there will also be signs of shock including pallor, sweating, weakness, and faintness. If you experience symptoms of this kind in pregnancy or when pregnancy is possible you should get help immediately as it is potentially a life-threatening situation.

Endometriosis—endometrial cells which normally line the wall of the uterus are sometimes found outside the uterus, generally in the pelvic cavity. The cells bleed but have no outlet. Adhesions may form causing pain and sometimes prevent conception.

Estrogen—A group of hormones essential for normal sexual development and healthy functioning of the reproductive system.

Fibroids—benign growths of fibrous connective tissue and muscle that develop within the wall of the uterus and can sometimes interfere with the implantation of an embryo.

Gonadotropins—hormones that stimulate activity in the ovaries and testes. They are essential for fertility and include follicle-stimulating hormone (FSH) and luteinizing hormones (LH).

Hyperprolactinemia—raised levels of the hormone prolactin; it can result in infertility.

Hypogonadism—underactivity of the testes or ovaries (gonads). It may be caused by disorders of the gonads or the pituitary gland resulting in deficiencies of gonadotrophic hormones. It causes deficiency of androgen in men and estrogen in women.

Hypothalamus—the hypothalamus is a gland within the brain which controls the sympathetic nervous system and also releases nerve signals which are converted by the pituitary gland into hormones. If the hypothalamus is failing to function correctly it can affect the glands of the endocrine system including the pituitary, thyroid and adrenal glands, testes and ovaries.

Hysterosalpingogram—insertion of an opaque dye into the uterus via the cervix under X ray. It can show if the fallopian tubes are blocked; if they are not, the dye will spill out through them into the pelvic cavity.

ICSI—intracytoplasmic sperm injection. The insertion of a single sperm into an egg via a very fine needle under a microscope.

Laparoscopy—a method of examining the inside of the abdomen through a viewing instrument.

Leucopenia—low levels of white blood cells.

Miscarriage—loss of a pregnancy before 24 weeks.

Mucorrhea—excessive production of mucus.

Oligospermia—very few sperm are present.

Pelvic inflammatory disease (PID)—infection of the female reproductive organs. PID is a common cause of pelvic pain and can be sexually transmitted or follow miscarriage, termination of pregnancy or childbirth. Symptoms include abdominal pain or tenderness, fever, and irregular periods. Pain may be worse immediately after a period or sex. It may also cause a feeling of being unwell, backache, or vomiting.

Pituitary—master gland which produces hormones. It controls activities of the other endocrine glands, which are responsible for production of luteinizing and follicle-stimulating hormones (LH and FSH) in both men and women which stimulate the testes and the ovaries.

Polycystic ovary syndrome (PCOS)—syndrome where periods may become very irregular or stop. It may be associated with multiple cysts on the ovaries.

Progesterone—hormone essential for reproductive functioning. It is produced by the ovaries during the second half of the cycle and by the placenta during pregnancy.

Polycythemia—unusually large numbers of red blood cells in the blood.

Retrograde ejaculation—the valve at the base of the bladder fails to close during ejaculation so that semen is forced back into the bladder.

Retroverted uterus—the uterus is tilted backwards toward the rectum rather than forwards toward the vagina. It occurs in about 20 percent of women.

Superovulation—the stimulation of a woman's ovaries with drugs to produce more eggs that usual in a monthly cycle.

Thrombocytopenia—reduction of the number of platelet cells in the blood.

Thromboembolism—blockage of a blood vessel by a blood clot.

Varicocele—varicose vein in the scrotum.

Vascular—relating to the blood vessels.

INDEX

see also Chinese herbalism
herbal teas 130, 133
heroin 89
holistic treatment 108, 180
homeopathy 60, 127–8, 142–50, 180
hormone disorders 113, 131, 146
human chorionic gonadotrophin
(hCG) 42, 49, 50, 91
human menopausal gonadotropin
(hMG) 41–2, 49
hyperprolactinemia 45
hypnotherapy 27, 90, 93, 102, 128,
150–7, 166, 180
hypogonadism 69, 91
hysterosalpingogram (HSG) 134, 137
hysteroscopy 47

ICSI (intracytoplasmic sperm injection) 15, 18, 35, 36
immunological infertility 19
impotence 74
induction treatment 116
infection 16, 24, 120–21, 132–3
infecundity 12
infertility, causes of 16
insecticides 95–8, 100
iron 13, 81, 82–3, 87, 131
isolation 9, 29, 32, 55, 167
IUI (intrauterine insemination) 47, 54,
83, 127, 135
IVF (in vitro fertilization) 15, 17, 31,
47–52, 60, 83, 127, 156, 160
drugs 22–3, 37, 41, 47, 48–50
multiple births 44, 51

Japanese herbalism 141
laparoscopy 21–2, 47, 49, 53, 59–60,
104, 134, 136–7
laparotomy 22
lifestyle 10, 17–19, 26–7, 71, 108, 144, 168
LSD 89
luteal phase defects 37, 39
luteinizing hormone (LH) 20, 37, 42,
46, 49, 103, 165
lysine 79

macrobiotic diet 66–7
magnesium 81, 83, 128

male infertility:
alternative treatments 112–13, 130,
141
causes 16–19, 27
manufactured foods 65
marijuana 89
masculinization 22, 23
massage 120, 121
meaning, finding 57
medical treatments 9–11, 31–54
meditation 166
men:
aromatherapy oils for 121
chlamydia in 25
and drugs 90–1
emotional effects on 34
and heat 99–100
herbs for 132
occupation 100–1
supplements for 73–9
see also male infertility
menopause 35, 92, 163
artificial 49, 50
premature 50
mental block 27
menstruation 20, 27
heavy (menorragia) 81, 82, 119, 131,
133–4
irregular 84, 87, 88, 89, 113, 131, 160
painful 22, 81, 119, 132, 141, 158
and weight 84–7
methadone 89
micro-surgery 23
milk 95
mineral supplements 72–3, 104–5, 111
for men 73–6
for women 79–83
miscarriage 12, 83–4, 113, 168–9, 182
in assisted conception 11
and diet 70, 71
and drugs 39, 42, 89
and grief 31, 33
homeopathic treatment 127–8
and pesticides 96
reflexology and 158
and smoking 92–3
and tubal infertility 24
molar pregnancy 114

Also by Nicki Wesson

NATURAL MOTHERING

A Guide to Holistic Therapies for Pregnancy, Birth, and Early Childhood

Natural therapies can enhance every stage of pregnancy, ease discomfort during labor, and offer effective, gentle treatment for infants and children. This comprehensive guide anwers questions and provides readers with expert advice on using the most effective complementary therapies, including:

- Acupuncture
- Aromatherapy
- Bach flower remedies
- Cranial osteopathy
- Homeopathy
- Hypnotherapy
- Massage
- Medical herbalism
- Reflexology

Nicki Wesson addresses such problems as difficulty conceiving, recurrent miscarriages, morning sickness, fatigue, insomnia, stretch marks, and stress. Sections on labor, birth, and the postpartum stage describe the physiological processes at work and provide important information on avoiding routine orthodox medical interventions whenever possible. Chapters on breastfeeding and caring for your newborn round out this complete guide. ISBN 0-89281-733-X • 240 pages • $14.95 pb

---

This and other Inner Traditions/Healing Arts Press titles are available at many fine bookstores, or, to order directly from the publisher, please send check or money order payable to Inner Traditions for the total amount, plus $3.50 shipping for the first book and $1.00 for each additional book to:

Inner Traditions, P.O. Box 388, Rochester, VT 05767
Visit our web site at: www.InnerTraditions.com